Practical Genetics for the O

Practical Genetics
for the Ob-Gyn

W. Allen Hogge *MD, MA*
Professor, Department of Obstetrics, Gynecology and Reproductive Sciences
University of Pittsburgh/Magee-Womens Hospital
Pittsburgh, Pennsylvania

Aleksandar Rajkovic *MD, PhD*
Professor, Department of Obstetrics, Gynecology and Reproductive Sciences
University of Pittsburgh/Magee-Womens Hospital
Pittsburgh, Pennsylvania

Mc Graw Hill Education | Medical

New York   Chicago   San Francisco   Athens   London   Madrid
Mexico City   Milan   New Delhi   Singapore   Sydney   Toronto

Practical Genetics for the Ob-Gyn, First Edition

1 2 3 4 5 6 7 8 9 0   CTP/CTP   18 17 16 15 14

ISBN 978-0-07-179721-4
MHID 0-07-179721-1

This book was set in Minion Pro by MPS Limited.
The editors were Alyssa Fried and Regina Y. Brown.
The production supervisor was Catherine H. Saggese.
Production management was provided by Asheesh Ratra of MPS Limited.
China Translation & Printing Services, Ltd. was printer and binder.

This book is printed on acid-free paper.

Library of Congress Cataloging-in-Publication Data

Hogge, W. Allen, author.
    Practical genetics for the OB-GYN / W. Allen Hogge, Aleksandar Rajkovic.
        p. ; cm.
    Includes index.
    ISBN 978-0-07-179721-4 (pbk. : alk. paper)—ISBN 0-07-179721-1 (MHID : alk. paper)
    I. Rajkovic, Aleksandar, author. II. Title.
    [DNLM: 1.   Prenatal Diagnosis. 2.   Genetic Counseling. 3.   Genetic Phenomena.
    4.   Genital Diseases, Female—genetics. 5.   Pregnancy Complications–genetics.
    WQ 209]
    RG628
    618.3'2075—dc23
                                                                    2014003881

McGraw-Hill books are available at special quantity discounts to use as premiums and sales promotions, or for use in corporate training programs. To contact a representative please visit the Contact Us pages at www.mhprofessional.com.

This book is dedicated to our children: Marcus, Kelly, Joanna, Andrei, Gabriel, and Ada, who have made us humble and brought us joy.

Table of Contents

Part 1 Basic Genetic Principles

Part 2 Clinical Genetics in Obstetrics and Gynecology

Preface

Thirty years ago when the senior author entered the field of genetics, obstetrician-gynecologists had little need for genetic principles as part of their training or practice. However, in three short decades, genetics has become an integral part of all aspects of women's health care. Molecular techniques have replaced culturing for infectious diseases, and the diagnosis and management of cervical disease is based on molecular assessment of human papillomavirus typing. Prenatal diagnosis has expanded from testing for chromosomal abnormalities and a few biochemical disorders to direct gene mutation testing for a host of genetic conditions. Screening for genetic diseases can now be done directly on fetal DNA circulating in the maternal blood stream, and represents the first population-wide application of genomics to clinical care. What was once a specialty focused on rare diseases, affecting very few patients, is now the basis for understanding who is pre-disposed to disease, how an individual will respond to therapy, and what cancer treatment is best, based on tumor profiles. The field is changing so rapidly that even those with specialized training in genetics have difficulty keeping up with the newest findings that have implication for patient care.

Our goal in creating this book is simple: to provide a basic text that can serve as the foundation for an OB/GYN resident, or practicing OB/GYN in the genetic principles that will allow them to integrate genetics into their practice, and allow them to interpret new literature through the lens of these basic principles. In the field of genetics, or genomics as it is currently described, no textbook can expect to be current. At the time of writing this manuscript, the number of disease-causing genes was over 4000, with more than 100,000 different mutations described in these 4000 genes. It is estimated over 300 new disease-causing mutations are being reported annually. We present broad principles we expect will provide the reader with the basic skill set necessary for what must be lifelong learning in the field of genomics. Our format is simple: we provide an introductory case scenario and base our discussion on how the case should be managed. It is our hope this approach can serve as the foundation for our reader to learn the genetic principles necessary to build the knowledge base required for good patient care.

Acknowledgment

There are many people who deserve our thanks. Our mentors, Mitchell Golbus and Joe Leigh Simpson, were among the visionaries who saw the key role genetics would play in the specialty of obstetrics and gynecology, and sparked our enthusiasm to be reproductive geneticists. We thank our wives, Joan Hogge and Ana Malinow, for their support of our careers, and especially for putting up with the time we spent "working on the book." We are indebted to Drs Svetlana and Alexander Yatsenko for sharing their special expertise in molecular cytogenomics and laboratory genetics, respectively, and for helping with many of the figures used in those chapters. The inspiration for many of the cases discussed in the book came from our genetic counseling colleagues Michele Clemens, Deanna Steele, Abigail Peffer, Luanne Fraer, Beth Kladny, Mary Dunkle, and Darcy Thull, as well as our clinical genetics colleagues Dr Marta Kolthoff and Dr Neil Saller. Special thanks go to Adele Leibowitz who organized and prepared our various manuscripts into a coherent whole, and to our editor at McGraw-Hill, Alyssa Fried, who guided us through the conception and birth of this project. Finally, we thank the many residents and fellows who have provided feedback on what they needed to learn to incorporate genetics into their practice.

Basic Genetic Principles

Gene Structure and Function

Knowledge of the genetic basis of health and disease has increased dramatically in the last 20 years. The first draft of the sequence of the human genome was published in 2001, and the Human Genome Project was completed in 2003.[1,2] From this project has come a detailed map of genes and genetic markers and a clearer understanding of how genes function. The intent of this chapter is to provide a basic understanding of gene structure and function and a glossary of terms that should be helpful in incorporating genetic screening and testing into a practice of obstetrics and gynecology. For those interested in a more comprehensive resource on basic molecular genetics, we suggest either Gelehrter et al or Nussbaum et al.[3,4]

■ ORGANIZATION OF THE GENOME

Within the human nucleus are 3 billion base pairs of DNA, contained in which are approximately 25,000 to 30,000 genes. The DNA is tightly wrapped around proteins called histones to form what are termed nucleosomes. Nucleosomes are organized into solenoid structures and looped around a nonhistone protein scaffold to form chromatin, which makes up chromosomes. Each chromosome is composed of densely packed nontranscribed DNA located near the centromere (heterochromatin), and less densely packed and transcribed DNA (euchromatin). Chapter 2 provides a more detailed discussion of the structure of chromosomes.

About three-quarters of the genome is unique, single-copy DNA, and the remaining one-quarter is made up of various forms of repetitive DNA. Less than 10% of the genome encodes genes. Initially, it was thought that the repetitive DNA, and much of the single-copy DNA, had no function. However, recent studies suggest that this "noncoding" DNA may be where the various "switches" are located that control gene function. Although more than 99% of DNA is identical in all humans, the small variations, known as polymorphisms, have been key to understanding the genetic basis of many diseases thought to have a genetic component, such as heart disease, diabetes, and other adult-onset disorders.

In addition to the nuclear genome, each cell contains a mitochondrial genome, approximately 16,500 nucleotides in length. The mitochondrial genome contains 37 genes, and these genes encode 13 essential mitochondrial proteins, 22 transfer RNAs (tRNAs), and 2 ribosomal RNAs (rRNAs). The mitochondria genome does not encode all of the proteins that make up mitochondria; the remaining proteins are encoded by the nuclear genome. Each mitochondrion usually contains multiple copies of mitochondrial DNA, and each healthy cell consists of several hundred mitochondria. If all the mitochondria in a given cell contain the same DNA sequence, this is called homoplasmy, while populations of mitochondria with differing DNA sequences give rise to heteroplasmy.

■ GENE STRUCTURE

Each gene is a unique series of four purine (adenine, guanine) and pyrimidine (thymine, cytosine) bases. The nucleotides that make up these genes are composed of a base, a phosphate, and a sugar moiety that polymerize into long polynucleotide chains. In the human genome, these polynucleotide chains form the double helix, and range in size from approximately 50 million base pairs (chromosome 21) to 250 million base pairs (chromosome 1, the largest chromosome). Individual genes themselves vary in size from as little as 1000 base pairs up to 2 million base pairs (the dystrophin gene on the X chromosome).

Genes are composed of one or more exons, which are the DNA sequences that are transcribed into messenger RNA (mRNA) that will be translated into a polypeptide at the ribosomal level. In addition to the exons, the gene has introns or intervening sequences that may transcribe RNA, but that RNA is not part of the mature mRNA that is found in the cytoplasm. The regions upstream and downstream to the exons are called the 5′ untranslated region and the 3′ untranslated region, respectively. These adjacent nucleotide sequences provide the molecular signals for "starting" and "stopping" the synthesis of mRNA. At the 5′ end of the gene is located the promoter region, which has the sequence necessary for the initiation of transcription. Within this region are several other DNA elements that are conserved among many different genes and play key roles in gene regulation. Within the 3′ untranslated end of the gene lies a region of DNA that contains a signal for the addition of a sequence of 100 to 200 adenosine bases (the poly A tail) to the end of the mature mRNA. Within both the 5′ and 3′ untranslated regions are many other regulating elements (enhancers, silencers, locus control regions) that

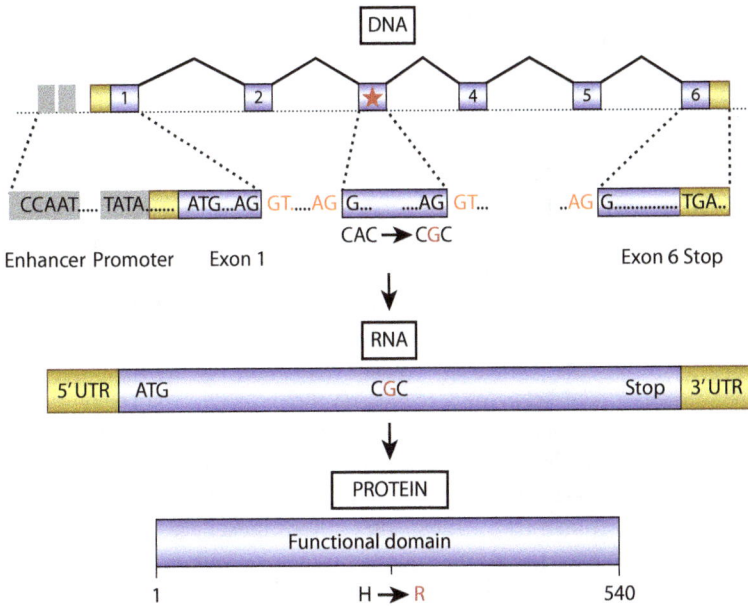

FIGURE 1-1. General elements of a typical human gene and its associated products. A six-exon gene is shown with upstream regulatory regions, such as promoters (TATA box, CCAAT box) in grey. Exons are composed of regions that do not encode protein (untranslated regions [UTR], depicted in yellow), and coding regions are shown in blue. The red star depicts a gene mutation that changes the nucleotide sequence from CAC to CGC, which translates into amino acid change from histidine (H) to arginine (R). This is an example of a missense mutation. The splice donor site includes a conserved dinucleotide sequence, GT, at the 5' end of the intron, while the splice acceptor site at the 3' end of the intron contains a conserved dinucleotide AG (highlighted in orange). Mutations within conserved splice donor and acceptor sites will cause abnormal splicing, and result in abnormal protein products.

are essential for gene expression and may be sites of mutation that cause genetic diseases by interfering with gene expression. Figure 1-1 illustrates a typical human gene and its associated products.

■ OVERVIEW OF GENE EXPRESSION

Initiation of the transcription of a gene is under the influence of transcription factors (specific proteins that function to "turn on" genes) that interact with promoters and other regulating elements. Transcription begins in a transcriptional "start site" on chromosomal DNA upstream from the coding DNA. Transcription continues through both exons and introns and past the coding sequences. Synthesis of the mRNA for coding proteins is done by RNA polymerase II, and proceeds from the 5′ to the 3′ end of the RNA. This means the DNA strand of the gene being transcribed is being read in the 3′ to 5′ direction.

One of the important promoter sequences is known as the "TATA box." It is a region, conserved in many genes, that is rich in adenine and thymine bases and is just upstream, by 25 to 30 base pairs, of the transcription start sites. It appears to be key in determining the position of the start of transcription. A second conserved region (CCAAT) is called the "CAT box." It is a few dozen base pairs farther upstream than the TATA box and is a key element in the expression of genes that are tissue specific. In the so-called "housekeeping genes", that are constitutively expressed in most tissues, these elements may be lacking in the promoter region. Rather, these housekeeping genes have promoter regions, rich in cytosines and guanines, that are referred to as CpG islands. These CG-rich sequences are thought to serve as binding sites for specific transcription factors.

Once the mRNA has been transcribed, a chemically modified guanine nucleotide (called a cap) is added to the 5′ end to prevent the mRNA from being degraded. Cleavage at a specific point on the 3′ end, downstream of the coding area, occurs, and a poly A tail is added to the 3′ end of the mRNA. This posttranscriptional modification takes place in the nucleus, as does RNA splicing, which removes RNA transcribed from introns. The mature mRNA must have only the transcripts of the exons to be a functional mRNA.

The splicing reactions are guided by specific DNA sequences at both the 5′ (splice donor sites) and 3′ ends (splice acceptor sites) of introns. The 5′ sequence, located immediately adjacent to the splice site, appears invariant among all genes. In similar fashion, there are key elements at the 3′ end. For example, in the β-globin splice reaction, the 3′ sequence consists of approximately 12 nucleotides, of which two are AG nucleotides located immediately 5′ to the intron/exon boundary, and appear essential for normal splicing.

The fully processed mRNA is then transported to the cytoplasm, where translation takes place. Because genes may contain more than one promoter or have alternative splice sites, the same gene may encode many different protein products. The concept of "one gene, one protein" is no longer valid.

In the cytoplasm, mRNA is translated into proteins by the action of tRNAs, each of which is specific for a particular amino acid. These tRNA molecules transfer the correct amino acid to their position on the mRNA template, resulting in a polypeptide chain. The key to translation is a code that identifies a specific amnio acid. This code is a combination of three adjacent bases along the mRNA, termed a codon. With four bases to create the three-base codon, there are 64 possible triplet combinations, known as the genetic code. Because there are only 20 amino acids, and 64 possible codons, most amino acids are coded by more than one codon. Only methionine and tryptophan are each specified by a single unique codon. Three of the codons are called "stop" codons because they designate termination of translation of the mRNA at that point. Of note, translation is always initiated at a codon specifying methionine (AUG), which is termed the initiation codon. This establishes the reading frame whereby each subsequent codon is read to determine the amino acid sequence. Although methionine is the first encoded amino acid always, it is usually removed before protein synthesis is completed.

■ OTHER MODIFIERS OF GENE EXPRESSION

Gene expression also can be controlled by what is termed epigenetic modification, which involves methylation of genes or modification of histone structures. Epigenetic modifications are essential for cells with otherwise identical DNA sequences to differentiate into specialized cells. Methylation of a gene's regulatory region prevents gene transcription and, thus, turns off the gene. This type of modification allows either tissue-specific gene activation or suppression. For example, globin genes are methylated in nonerythroid tissues, but unmethylated in cells like reticulocytes that must produce hemoglobin. Some genes are essential to early human development but would be detrimental after the embryonic period of life. Methylation and demethylation are, therefore, essential to the temporal control of genes that function in early embryonic development. That certain genes may demonstrate different methylation, depending on the parent of origin, is the biological basis for the imprinting disorders discussed in Chapter 2.

In addition to methylation effects, there are multiple potential modifications of histone proteins that can activate or suppress gene expression. Specific enzymes can acetylate, phosphorylate, methylate, or ubiquitinate histones, which can alter gene expression, DNA repair processes, or chromosomal condensation.

■ GENETIC VARIATION: MUTATIONS OR POLYMORPHISMS

As noted earlier, the sequence of nuclear DNA is more than 99% identical between any two humans. The small fraction of variability in DNA is responsible for the genetically determined differences among humans. Some DNA sequence changes have little or no effect, and others result in significant medical disorders. Between these two extremes are the many DNA sequence changes that provide the significant phenotypic variability that results in physical differences, differing susceptibilities to disease, variation in response to medications, and the myriad of differences between humans. However, for purposes of this book we will focus on those types of changes that result in, or predispose to disease.

Mutations can be defined as changes in the nucleotide sequence, or arrangement, of DNA. This broad definition would include changes in chromosome numbers, such as in Down syndrome, or changes in chromosome structure, such as an unbalanced translocation, as mutations. We have chosen to define "mutation" more narrowly as an alteration in an individual gene. By this definition, a mutation is defined as a change in the DNA sequence that may be as little as a single nucleotide or affect many thousands of base pairs, but one that always involves a single gene. There is no correlation between the size of the sequence change, and the phenotypic effects. A single nucleotide change in the coding sequence of a given gene may lead to complete loss of gene function or to the formation of a variant protein with altered properties. The best clinical example of the single-nucleotide change is sickle cell disease.

Gene mutations, which include base pair substitutions, insertions, and deletions, originate either through errors in DNA replication, or from failure to repair DNA damage. Most replication errors are recognized and corrected by a series of DNA repair enzymes. The overall mutation rate from replication errors is only 10^{-10} per base pair per cell division.[4] Mutations from failure to repair DNA damage are caused by chemical processes such as depurination, demethylation, or deamination. Unless repair is effected by the various DNA repair enzymes, these will remain as permanent mutations.

Types of Gene Mutations

Mutations can range from a single-base pair change to deletion of millions of base pairs. Mutations are the basis of population diversity, but may also be the cause of serious genetic disorders. In the context of clinical genetics, the term "mutation" is reserved for those gene changes that result in significant phenotypic manifestations.

Nucleotide substitution can be a single nucleotide change, called a point mutation. Such an alteration in the DNA sequence can modify a codon to cause a change from one amino acid to another in the protein product. Because these mutations alter the "sense" of the coding strand of DNA, resulting in a different amino acid, they are called missense mutations. Missense mutations account for over half of all mutations that cause human genetic disorders. Single-base changes in areas such as the promoter region may not alter protein structure, but by changing gene expression, they may result in a significantly diminished amount of protein product.

RNA splicing mutations that are near the intron/exon boundary in key nucleotide sequences can abolish normal RNA splicing and result in specific genetic diseases. Alternatively splicing mutations can occur because of a base substitution in an intron, creating new splice sites in the gene, again resulting in an abnormal protein with phenotypic consequences.

Small deletions or insertions of base pairs that are not multiples of 3 and that occur in a coding sequence, will alter the normal reading frame, resulting in a different sequence of amino acids. These mutations are called frame-shift mutations. Even if there is not a frame-shift mutation, the addition or loss of base pairs can lead to loss of, or addition of, an amino acid to the protein, which can alter its function and result in a genetic disease. Approximately one-quarter of all mutations causing human disease are due to addition or loss of only a few base pairs.

Trinucleotide repeat mutations are more fully discussed in subsequent chapters, but in brief, these mutations are the result of an expansion in an area of repeating nucleotide triplets that are normally found in some areas of the genome. These areas may be in the coding region or in the transcribed, but untranslated, region. An expansion of the repeat in a coding area is likely to generate an abnormal protein, while an expansion in the transcribed, but untranslated, region may interfere with either transcription or mRNA processing.

As sequencing of the human genome has become more commonplace, many other types of mutations are being discovered and other mechanisms leading to genetic disease elucidated. Subsequent chapters will provide more detail on how these mutations result in genetic conditions seen in the practice of obstetrics and gynecology.

New mutations are most easily recognized in the population by the birth of a child with a "new to the family" autosomal dominant or X-linked fully penetrant genetic disorder, such as achondroplasia or Duchenne muscular dystrophy. From studies with these families, we know the median gene mutation rate to be approximately 1×10^{-6} mutations per locus per generation. Because most errors occur during DNA replication, and males have many more DNA replications during sperm formation than females in egg formation, most new genetic mutations are paternal in origin. There is also an increase in the incidence of new dominant mutations with increasing paternal age.

Polymorphisms are the minor changes in DNA sequence that differ between individuals, and make up the 0.1% variation between humans. Some of this variation is within genes themselves, and these different forms of the same gene are referred to as alleles. For example, in discussing genetic diseases, the normally functional gene is called the "wild-type" or "normal" allele, and there may be several mutated forms of gene, each defined as a mutant allele. By convention, if an allele occurs in more than 1% of the population, it is called a genetic polymorphism. Those that are seen in less than 1% of the population are designated as rare variants. Depending on how gene function is altered by the specific mutation, the severity of the disease produced can vary based on the specific allele inherited.

One of the outcomes of the Human Genome Project was the finding that there are single nucleotide changes, occurring approximately every 200 to 500 base pairs, that in most cases, appear to be benign changes, and do not affect gene function. These *single nucleotide polymorphisms* are useful genetic markers that have been key to understanding the genetic component of many adult-onset disorders.

As sequencing has become more common place multiple variants in DNA sequence have been found, many of which are benign changes and are called benign variants. On the other hand, some of the variants, also known as pathogenic variants, modify gene function, resulting in consistent phenotypic changes and leading to a host of syndromes. Finally, variants are often detected that have not been previously reported, and these changes are called *variants of unknown significance*. As more cases are published or entered into national databases, these variants will be reclassified as either benign or pathologic. Databases that harbor human sequences and contain well phenotyped individuals are essential to differentiate between benign and pathogenic variants. Animal models of human gene variants also are very important tools for understanding the function of genes and their variation. These animal models include zebrafish, mice, and primates, and often rely on transgenic technologies to modify the genome.

GLOSSARY

Allele: Alternative form of a gene; a single allele for each locus is inherited from each patient.

Base pair (bp): A pair of complementary nucleotide bases, as in double-stranded DNA. Used as the unit of measurement of the length of a DNA sequence.

Cap: A modified nucleotide added to the 5′ end of a growing mRNA chain, required for normal processing, stability, and translation of mRNA.

Chromatin: An intranuclear and intrachromosomal complex made up of DNA, and histone and nonhistone proteins that condense to form chromosomes during cell division.

Codon: A section of DNA (three nucleotide pairs in length) that codes for a single amino acid.

DNA methylation: A process for control of tissue specific gene expression. Methylation "turns off" the regulatory region of a gene, thereby preventing DNA transcription.

Epigenetic: Inherited changes in phenotype or gene expression that are caused by mechanisms other than changes in the underlying DNA sequence (eg, by methylation).

Exon: A region of a gene made up of DNA sequences that will be transcribed into mRNA.

Frame-shift: A mutation caused by deletions or insertions that are not a multiple of 3 base pairs. Results in a change in the reading frame by which triplet codons are translated into protein.

Gene: A unit of heredity responsible for the inheritance of a specific trait that occupies a fixed chromosomal site and corresponds to a sequence of nucleotides along a DNA molecule.

Genome: The entire complement of genetic material in a chromosome set.

Genomic imprinting: The phenomenon by which certain genes are expressed in a parent-of-origin specific manner. Imprinted genes are expressed only from the allele inherited from the mother or the father.

Hereditary unstable DNA (triplet repeat expansion): Gene containing a region of triplet-codon repeats such as $(CGG)_n$. The number of triplet repeats can increase during meiosis. If the expansion of repeats reaches a critical number, the gene becomes methylated and is turned off, resulting in phenotypic abnormalities.

Heterochromatin: Chromatin that remains condensed throughout interphase. It contains DNA that is genetically inactive and replicates late in the S phase of the cell cycle.

Intron: The region of a gene that is made up of noncoding DNA sequences and lies between the exons.

Locus: The position occupied by a gene on a chromosome. Different forms of the gene (*alleles*) may occupy the locus.

Missense: A mutation that alters a codon so that it encodes a different amino acid.

Mitochondrial inheritance: The inheritance of a trait encoded on the mitochondrial genome. Because mitochondria are inherited exclusively from the mother, mitochondrial inheritance is exclusively maternal.

Mutation: An alteration of DNA sequences in a gene that result in a heritable change in protein structure or function that frequently has adverse effects.

Nonsense mutation: A single-based substitution in DNA resulting in a chain-termination codon.

Nucleotide: A component of a DNA or RNA molecule composed of a nitrogenous base, one deoxyribose or ribose sugar, and one phosphate group. In DNA, adenine specifically joins to thymine and guanine joins to cytosine. In RNA, uracil replaces thymine.

Point mutation: A single nucleotide base-pair change in DNA.

Polyadenylation site: In the synthesis of mature mRNA, a site at which a sequence of 20 to 200 adenosine residues (the poly A tail) is added to the 3′ end of an RNA transcript, aiding its transport out of the nucleus and, usually, its stability.

Polymorphisms: The occurrence in the same population of more than one allele or genetic marker at the same locus.

Promoter: A DNA sequence located in the 5′ end of a gene at which transcription is initiated.

Reading frame: One of the 3 possible ways of reading a nucleotide sequence as a series of triplets. An *open reading frame* contains no termination codons and thus is potentially translatable into protein.

RNA polymerase: An enzyme that synthesizes RNA on a DNA template.

Silencer (repressor) DNA: DNA sequences located upstream or downstream of a gene that can increase and decrease transcriptional activity of the gene.

Single nucleotide polymorphism: DNA sequence variations that occur when a single nucleotide (A, T, C, or G) in the genome sequence is altered.

Splicing: The splicing out of introns and splicing together of exons in the generation of mature mRNA from the primary transcript.

TATA box: A consensus sequence in the promoter region of many genes that is located about 25 base pairs upstream from the start site of transcription and that determines the start site.

Termination codon: One of the 3 codons (UAG, UAA, and UGA) that terminate synthesis of a polypeptide. Also called a *stop codon.*

Transcription: The process of RNA synthesis from a DNA template that is directed by RNA polymerase.

Translation: The synthesis of a polypeptide from its mRNA template.

REFERENCES

1. International Human Genome Sequencing Consortium. Initial sequencing and analysis of the human genome. *Nature.* 2001;409:860-921.

2. International Human Genome Sequencing Consortium. Finishing the euchromatic sequence of the human genome. *Nature.* 2004;431:931-945.

3. Gelehrter TD, Collins FS, Ginsburg D. *Principles of Medical Genetics.* 2nd ed. Baltimore, MD: Williams & Wilklins; 1997.

4. Nussbaum RL, McInnes RR, Willard HF. *Genetics in Medicine.* Philadelphia, PA: Saunders Elsevier; 2007.

Organization and Structure of Human Chromosomes

The human genome is comprised of nuclear DNA sequences, tightly packed into distinct subunits called chromosomes and hundreds to thousands of circular DNA molecules within the mitochondrion. DNA sequences that encode for proteins account for few percent of the total genome, and the rest of the genome is involved in coding for various RNA molecules that do not code for protein (noncoding RNA) as well as regulatory function. DNA packed into chromosomes is coated with histone and nonhistone proteins, and these proteins play an important role in the regulation of gene expression. There are a total of 22 autosomal

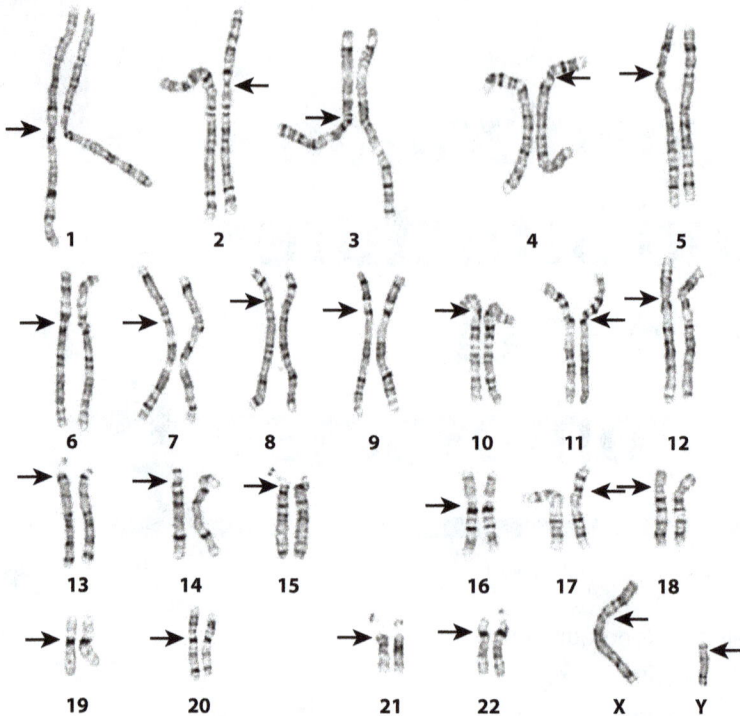

FIGURE 2-1. **A human normal male karyotype.** Homologous chromosomes (homologues), the two chromosomes in a pair of autosomes, are composed of similar (but not identical) DNA sequences. Each homologue encodes the same set of genes in the same order, but may contain different variant form of the same gene (allele), as well as variable noncoding DNA (introns). Centromeres are indicated by arrows, separating the short and long arms.

chromosomes (1-22) and the sex-determining X and Y chromosomes (Figure 2-1). The gametes, eggs and sperm, each contain a haploid set of 23 different chromosomes that upon fertilization gives rise to the diploid set, 46 chromosomes. In a normal diploid human cell, 23 chromosome pairs are present: 22 pairs of autosomes and two sex chromosomes—XX in females and XY in males. In each individual, each member of a pair is derived from either the father or the mother.

Chromosomes must be replicated at high fidelity and separated into their daughter cells with each cell division. Centromeres and telomeres are important specialized DNA structures on chromosomes. DNA replication during the interphase stage of mitosis produces two copies of a chromosome (sister chromatids) that are connected at the centromere (Figures 2-1 and 2-2). The kinetochore, a complex of proteins that interact with the centromere, serves as the attachment point for the spindle fibers during cell division and enable separation of sister chromatids into individual cells. Chromosome fragments that lack a centromere (acentric fragments) do not become attached to the spindle, and fail to be included in the nuclei

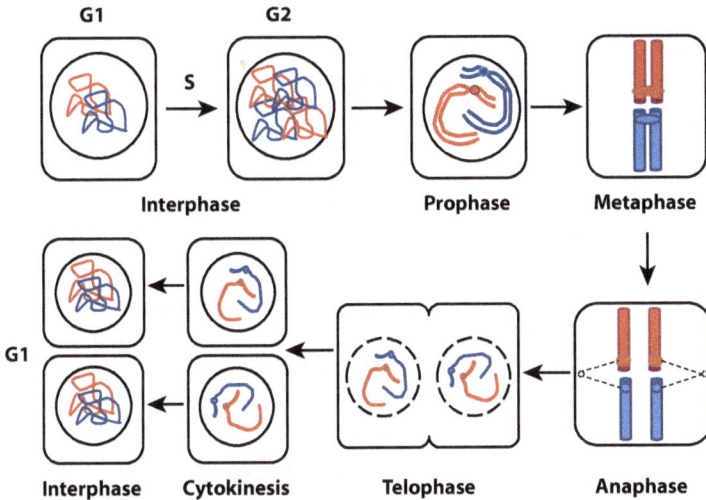

FIGURE 2-2. The cell cycle. For most cells, interphase accounts for about 90% of the cell cycle in which the cell grows, matures, and carries out its life function. Interphase has three stages: G1, S, and G2. During the G1 stage, each chromosome contains only one (unreplicated) molecule of DNA. The chromatin is diffuse within the nucleus. Extracellular growth factors stimulate cell proliferation to S stage in which the cell replicates its DNA. At the end of the S stage each chromosome contains two chromatids, and after the S phase, the cell enters G2 and is ready for mitosis. Mitosis is composed of four stages: prophase, metaphase, anaphase and telophase, resulting in division of the nucleus. The cytoplasm of the parental cell divides into two daughter cells during cytokinesis, and the chromosomes begin to decondense while the two new daughter cells enter the G1 phase.

of the daughter cells. Telomeres are located at the end of each chromosome, are composed of DNA and protein complexes and serve as caps to maintain chromosome integrity and to prevent chromosomes from fusing and from degradation. The telomere consists of a simple 5'-TTAGGG-3' sequence that is repeated thousands of times. With each round of DNA replication in a somatic cell, telomeres are shortened and finally lost, providing a mechanism for natural aging and death.[1]

■ MEIOSIS

Meiosis is a specialized cell division that generates haploid gametes ready for fertilization, and consists of meiosis I and meiosis II. Meiosis I, also known as a reductional division, reduces the number of chromosomes from 46 (92 chromatids) to 23 (46 chromatids), The sister chromatids will separate and segregate to daughter cells during meiosis II to produce four haploid cells containing 23 chromosomes. Meiosis I prophase is the most unique aspect of meiosis and is composed of leptotene, zygotene, pachytene, diplotene, and diakinesis stages. During the first four stages homologues pair, and recombine. In a female, meiosis I commences during first trimester in utero and arrests in diplotene stage of meiosis I, prior to the formation of primordial follicles (circa 20 weeks of gestation). Meiosis I in females resumes after puberty in response to hormonal stimulation. Meiosis II completion requires fertilization. In males, meiosis I commences at the time of puberty, and spermatogonial stem cells continue to supply male gonads with spermatocytes that continually enter meiosis to generate haploid spermatozoa. Females on the other hand do not have comparable stem cells and are born with a finite pool of oocytes that is significantly depleted by age 30 and only a few oocytes remain by the time of menopause (51 years of age).

In oogenesis, after the first meiotic division, two daughter cells greatly differ in size. A large secondary oocyte enters meiosis II, while a small cell (polar body) degenerates. A second polar body is produced after fertilization and completion of the second meiotic division. In females, one oocyte gives rise to one mature egg for fertilization and two polar bodies, while one spermatocyte gives rise to four spermatozoa.

Meiotic Nondisjunction

Meiotic chromosome segregation errors increase dramatically with maternal age. Meiosis I errors are the predominant cause of aneuploidy (80%-90%) (Figure 2-3). Although pregnancy loss can occur at any gestational age, most conceptions are clinically unrecognized pregnancies in which a fertilized egg fails to implant in the

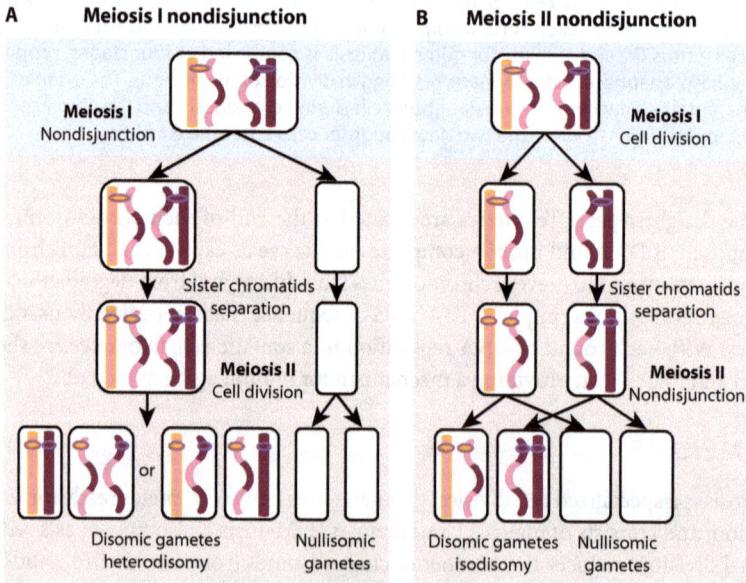

FIGURE 2-3. Nondisjunction in meiosis. (A) Abnormal segregation of homologous chromosomes during the first meiosis division results in formation of disomic and nullisomic gametes, containing both maternal and paternal chromosomes (heterodisomy) and missing a chromosome, respectively. Heterodisomy is determined by the origin of the centromere and the pericentromeric regions, as DNA sequences near centromeres are rarely involved in meiotic crossing over. **(B)** As a result of nondisjunction during meiosis II disomic and nullisomic gametes are produced, however disomic gametes contain only paternal or only maternal chromosomes (isodisomy).

uterus, or a pregnancy is lost shortly after implantation (biochemical pregnancy).[2,3] Meiotic nondisjunction is usually a random error in the oocyte or sperm and, therefore, the recurrence risk is approximately 1%. However, some couples may carry a genetic predisposition for nondisjunction due to mutations in genes that regulate meiosis, and they will suffer higher rates of recurrent miscarriages and aneuploid pregnancies. In other couples that have recurrence of aneuploidy with the same chromosome, germline mosaicism may be the cause. Germline mosaicism, also known as gonadal mosaicism, means that a subset of germ cells is genetically abnormal. The risk of transmission will depend on the percent of affected germ cells in the gonad. In approximately 5% of young couples with a previous child with Down syndrome, one of the parents will have germline mosaicism for trisomy 21.[4,5]

Uniparental Disomy

Uniparental disomy (UPD) is a condition in which both homologues of a chromosome or a chromosome segment are inherited from only one parent. UPD is encountered in approximately 1:3500 newborns. In general, it requires two independent nondisjunction events to produce UPD. As a result of nondisjunction during meiosis I, both chromosomes are transmitted to an egg or sperm (Figure 2-3A). These disomic gametes have a pair of nonidentical chromosomes (nonidentical due to recombination) originated from the two homologues (heterodisomy). In contrast, errors in meiosis II result in isodisomy, due to a nondisjunction of sister chromatids (Figure 2-3B). Fertilization of the disomic gametes would result in trisomy; however, loss of one of the three chromosomes early in mitosis (trisomy or embryo rescue) can lead to UPD (Figure 2-4). UPD may also occur as a result of a monosomy rescue, when a nullisomic gamete is fertilized by a normal haploid gamete, or when a normal zygote loses a chromosome due to mitotic nondisjunction. A single parental homologue is replicated postzygotically, leading to whole chromosome isodisomy. UPD can involve an entire chromosome or a segment (segmental UPD). UPD is classified as maternal (mat) or paternal (pat), depending on the origin of the disomic chromosome. It is further classified as uniparental heterodisomy or uniparental isodisomy.[6] In approximately 70% of UPD cases the karyotype is normal, while in 30% of patients UPDs are seen in association with numerical or structural chromosomal abnormalities.[7]

UPD caused by isodisomy is associated with an increased risk for a recessive disorder, while heterodisomy for the majority of chromosomes does not cause health problems. A few chromosomes (6, 7, 11, 14, 15, and 20) contain genes and regulatory elements that are differentially expressed depending on whether the chromosome was inherited from the father or mother. If a paternal or maternal imprinted chromosome is missing due to UPD, the individual will be affected with one of the various imprinting disorders (Table 2-1). As an example, Prader-Willi syndrome is caused by a deletion of the 15q12 region on the paternal chromosome or by maternal UPD (due to absence of paternal chromosome 15).

The diagnosis of UPD requires molecular testing. Microarrays containing SNP probes allow genotype analysis and can detect long contiguous regions with homozygosity (absence of heterozygosity or AOH) suggestive of identical DNA

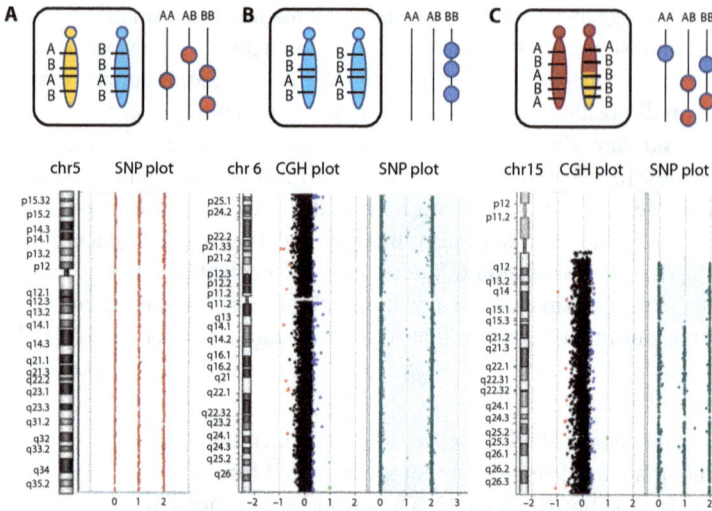

FIGURE 2-4. UPD detection using CGH+SNP microarray. (A) Top, schematic representation of a cell with a normal biparental inheritance, showing a pair of homologous chromosomes inherited from both parents. The genotype of four alleles is shown. Genotypes AA, AB, and BB are distributed randomly along a chromosome. Below, the SNP plot shows normal allele distribution for chromosome 5. In a CGH + SNP microarray, SNPs probes are designed to include the enzymes recognition sites. After restriction digestion and array hybridization, SNP probes produce the low "0," intermediate "1," and high "2" fluorescent signal intensity, corresponding to the AA, AB, and BB allele, respectively. Red dots (SNP probes) are randomly distributed between the 0, 1, and 2 lines consistent with biparental inheritance. **(B)** Top, schematic representation of uniparental isodisomy. Both homologous chromosomes are identical and inherited from one of the parents. Below, results of CGH + SNP microarray analysis in a patient with neonatal diabetes mellitus. The CGH plot shows a normal DNA copy number for chromosome 6 (disomy). The SNP plot shows an absence of heterozygous AB alleles for the entire chromosome 6 consistent with uniparental inheritance. **(C)** Top, schematic representation of segmental UPD. Two homologous chromosomes are identical at the proximal region but are distinct at the distal portion of a chromosome as a result of a meiotic recombination. Bottom, CGH + SNP analysis of a patient with Prader-Willi syndrome. The CGH analysis is consistent with normal DNA copy number for chromosome 15, but the SNP plot detected segmented UPD for the proximal 15q, as well as a normal allele distribution for the rest of chromosome 15.

sequences. The presence of AOH regions on a single chromosome is consistent with uniparental isodisomy (Figure 2-4). SNP-containing microarrays can identify isodisomy, but they are unable to detect whole chromosome uniparental heterodisomy. Although both chromosomes are inherited from the same parent, they are not identical, so genotype comparison between the child and parent is required to detect uniparental heterodisomy.

Multiple constitutional regions of homozygosity on the same chromosome may represent UPD and can be confirmed by methylation analysis of the imprinted genes, microsatellite or microarray SNP genotype analysis of parental and patient samples. In contrast, multiple AOH regions on multiple chromosomes are characteristic of consanguineous relationship (Figure 2-5).

■ **TABLE 2-1.** Imprinting Disorders

Chromosome	UPD	Syndrome	OMIM
6	upd(6)pat	Transient neonatal diabetes, TND	#601410
7	upd(7)mat	Silver-Russell syndrome, SRS	#180860
11	upd(11)pat	Beckwith-Wiedemann syndrome, BWS	#130650
11	upd(11)mat	Silver-Russell syndrome, SRS	#180860
14	upd(14)pat	Paternal UPD(14) syndrome	#608149
14	upd(14)mat	Temple syndrome, TS	None
15	upd(15)pat	Angelman syndrome, AS	#105830
15	upd(15)mat	Prader-Willi syndrome, PWS	#176270
20	upd(20)pat	Pseudohypoparathyroidism type 1b	#103580

OMIM, online Mendelian inheritance in man. (www.ncbi.nlm.nih.gov/omim)

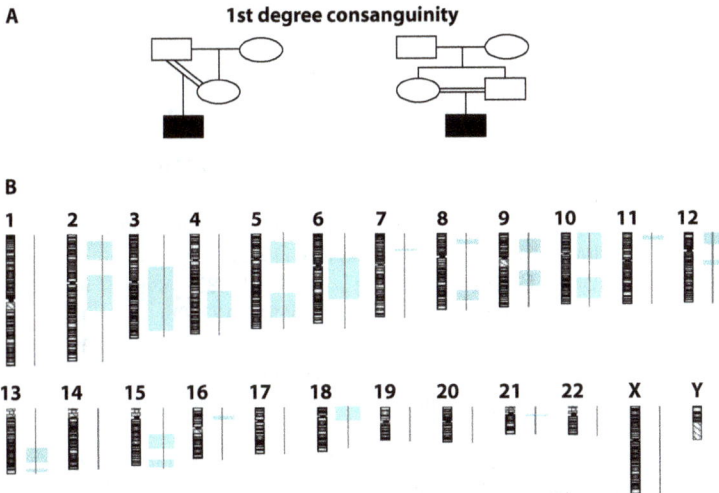

FIGURE 2-5. Detection of consanguinity by SNP-containing microarrays. (A) Pedigrees indicating a first degree relationship. (B) The CGH + SNP microarray analysis detected multiple contiguous regions with absence of heterozygosity (AOH) through whole-genome (light blue blocks), consistent with consanguinity.

Errors of Recombination

Homologous recombination causes DNA segments to exchange between homologous chromosomes during mitosis or meiosis. In mitosis, recombination is essential in proliferating cells to repair broken DNA. In meiosis, recombination promotes genetic diversity and proper homologous chromosome segregation. Errors in meiotic recombination can affect overall genome stability during gametogenesis and promote chromosome nondisjunction.

Meiotic recombination normally occurs between allelic sequences. However, recombination may also take a place between nonallelic DNA sequences that share

■ **TABLE 2-2.** Genomic Disorders

Location	Genomic Disorder Associated With Deletions	Genomic Disorder Associated With Duplications	Size, Mb
1q21.1	TAR region (OMIM 274000)	Not known	0.347-0.357
1q21.1	1q21.1 microdeletion (OMIM 612474)	1q21.1 microduplication (OMIM 612475)	1.19
2q13	Carrier juvenile nephronophthisis	Benign CNV	0.150
3q29	3q29 microdeletion syndrome (OMIM 609425)	3q29 microduplication syndrome (OMIM 611936)	1.6
7q11.23	Williams-Beuren syndrome (OMIM 194050)	WBS duplication syndrome (OMIM 609757)	1.5-1.8
15q11-q13	AS (OMIM 105830)/PWS (OMIM 176270)	15q11-q13 duplication syndrome (OMIM 608636)	0.50 to ~6.0
15q13	15q11-q13 deletion syndrome (CHRNA7) (OMIM 612001)	Unclear (CHRNA7) (OMIM 612001)	0.400 1.5-1.8
16p13.1	16p13.1 Microdeletion predisposing to autism and/or MR	16p13.1 Microduplication	1.3
16p11.2-p12	16p11.2 deletion syndrome (OMIM 613604)	Pathogenic—GCAD 23196	8.7
16p11.2	16p11.2 deletion syndrome (OMIM 611913)	16p11.2 duplication syndrome (OMIM 611913)	0.593-0.706
17p11.2	SMS (OMIM 182290)	PTLS (OMIM 610883)	3.7
17p12	HNPP (OMIM 162500)	CMT1A (OMIM 118220)	1.4
17q11.2	neurofibromatosis type I (OMIM 613675)	NF1 critical region microduplication syndrome	1.2-1.4
17q12	17q12 deletion syndrome (OMIM614527)	17q12 duplication syndrome (OMIM 614526)	1.5
17q23	17q23.1-q23.2 deletion syndrome (OMIM 613355)	17q23.1-q23.2 duplication syndrome (OMIM 613618)	2.1
22q11.21	DiGeorge/VCFS (OMIM 188400/192430)	Chromosome 22q11.2 microduplication (OMIM 608363)	1.5-3.0
22q11.23	22q11.2 Distal microdeletion (OMIM 611867)	Unclear	~2.5

high degree of homology. Repetitive elements that share high degree of homology in multiple locations in the genome can mediate genomic instability, causing chromosomal rearrangements such as deletions, duplications, inversions, and translocations. The nonallelic homologous recombination (NAHR) causes recurrent alterations in the human genome (genomic disorders), with pleiotropy of phenotypes including reproductive disorders. Deletions and duplications in the same chromosomal region may arise as a result of NAHR, leading to genomic disorders (Table 2-2). Genomic disorders are usually submicroscopic abnormalities, occur

TABLE 2-3. Organization and Structure of Human Chromosomes

Incidence of Common Chromosomal Disorders in Newborns	
Chromosome	Frequency at Birth
Pericentric inversion	1:100
Balanced translocation	1:500
Trisomy 21	1:700
47,XXY (Klinefelter)	1:1000 males
47,XYY	1:1000 males
47,XXX	1:1000 females
Unbalanced translocation	1:2000
45,X (Turner syndrome)	1:5000 females
Trisomy 18 (Edwards syndrome)	1:6000
Trisomy 13 (Patau syndrome)	1:10000

sporadically in the population, regardless of the parental age, and can be detected by chromosomal microarrays.[8,9]

TYPES AND MECHANISMS OF CHROMOSOME ABNORMALITIES

Chromosomal abnormalities include numerical aberrations (aneuploidy and polyploidy), structural balanced rearrangements (translocations, insertions and inversions), and unbalanced structural aberrations such as deletions, duplications, triplications, derivative, iso-, ring, and marker chromosomes, as well as complex rearrangements. Occasionally, chromosomal abnormalities are not changes in the number and structure, but result from epigenetic events such as UPD. The incidence of common chromosomal disorders in newborns is depicted in Table 2-3.

Numerical Chromosome Abnormalities

Aneuploidy occurs when a cell gains or loses chromosomes to cause tetrasomy, trisomy, monosomy, and nullisomy. In humans, aneuploidy is a common condition estimated to affect as many as 60% of all conceptions.[10] Nondisjunction is a failure of chromosome pairs to separate properly in germ cells during meiosis (meiotic nondisjunction) or after fertilization (mitotic nondisjunction) and leads to aneuploidy. Aneuploidy for all chromosomes has been reported in conceptuses, and generally results in spontaneous abortion for most, often before pregnancy is clinically recognized. About 5% of clinically recognized pregnancies are found to have aneuploidy.[11] Trisomy (three copies of a particular chromosome) is the most common type of aneuploidy and better tolerated by the conceptus than monosomy (chromosome loss). Fetuses with trisomy for chromosomes 13, 18, or 21 can survive to term, while other autosomal trisomies are rarely observed in live-born infants. Sex chromosome aneuploidy, such as 45,X; 47,XXX; 47,XXY;

and 47,XYY, is a frequent condition, found in 1:400 live births. Tetrasomy (four copies) and pentasomy (five copies) involving only the X chromosome have been observed, and the phenotype becomes more severe as the number of X chromosomes increases.

Aneuploidy may be present in a mosaic state when a chromosomal abnormality exists only in a subset of cells. Mosaic autosomal trisomy may be viable, depending on the tissues affected and the percent of abnormal cells. Mosaic trisomy 8, 9, and 14 are conditions associated with recognizable clinical syndromes.

Autosomal monosomies are usually incompatible with fetal survival, leading to early pregnancy losses. Only few cases of living newborns with apparently complete monosomy 21 have been reported.[12] Monosomy X (Turner syndrome) affects 1 in 500 newborn females; however, only 3% to 5% of fetuses with monosomy X survive to term.[13]

Polyploidy is a numerical chromosome abnormality where an extra haploid set of chromosomes is present. The most common form is triploidy or 69 chromosomes, which can contain different sex chromosome complements (69,XXX; 69,XXY; or 69,XYY) (Figure 2-6). In triploidy, two haploid sets from one parent and one haploid set from the other parent combine to form a zygote. The most common cause of triploidy is a fertilization of a haploid egg by two sperm (dispermy). Triploidy also can result from the fertilization of a normal haploid egg by a diploid sperm (diandric triploidy), or by the fertilization of a diploid egg by a normal haploid sperm (digynic triploidy). Triploidy accounts for approximately

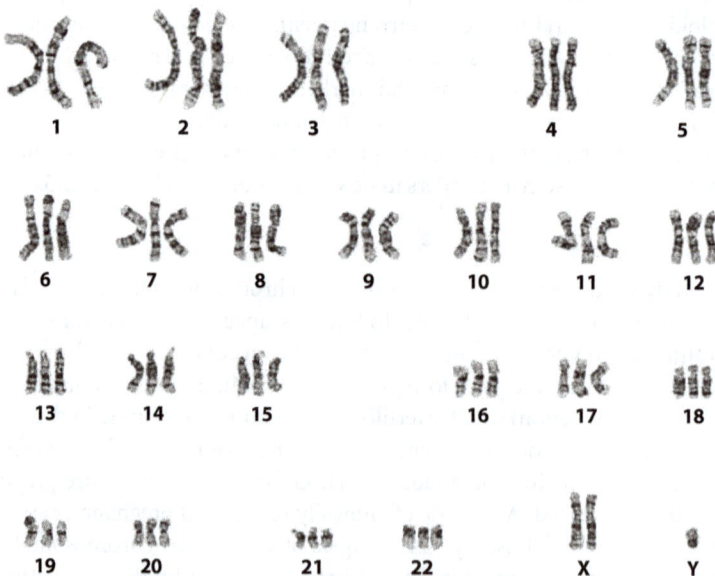

FIGURE 2-6. **G-banded karyotype showing triploidy.** A total of 69 chromosomes are shown. Each autosome has three homologous chromosomes, and three sex chromosomes (XXY) are present.

40% of early spontaneous pregnancy losses, while being seen in only 1% to 3% of recognized conceptions. Fetuses with mosaicism for diploid/triploid cells have also been observed among spontaneous abortuses, and some may survive to term. Tetraploidy, or 92 chromosomes, is a rare, usually nonviable condition, which may result from the failure of the cytokinesis after the first zygotic division (Figure 2-2). Very few fetuses and infants have been diagnosed with tetraploidy mosaicism.

Structural Chromosome Rearrangements

Structural abnormalities occur as a result of chromosomal breakage due to DNA damage or faulty DNA recombination. Abnormalities of chromosome structure can be either unbalanced or balanced and may result in birth defects, intellectual disability, and increased risk for infertility or pregnancy loss. Balanced structural rearrangements (Figure 2-7) are characterized by the transposition of chromosome segments to the wrong location (translocation and insertion), or changes in orientation or order (inversion), but there is no loss or gain of chromosomal material at the breakpoints. Unbalanced structural rearrangements (Figure 2-8) comprise abnormalities with gain or loss of significant amount of genetic material.

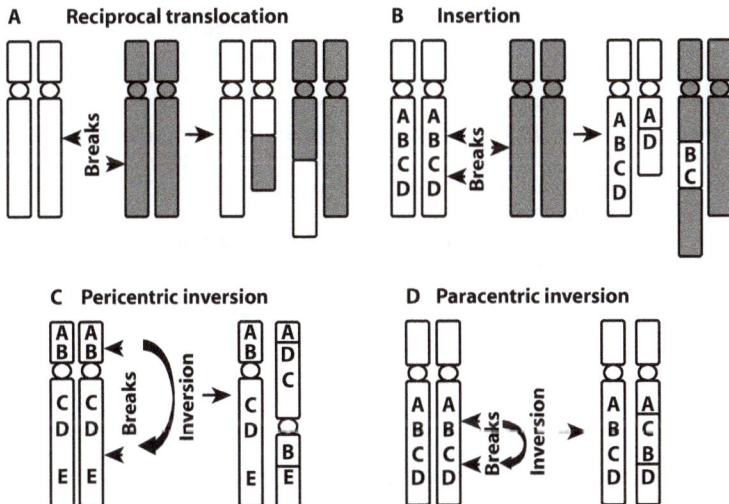

FIGURE 2-7. Schematic illustration of balanced chromosome rearrangements. (A) Reciprocal translocations can occur between nonhomologous chromosomes. Breaks in the DNA (arrowheads) at two different chromosomes, followed by exchange of chromosomal segments distal to the breaks, will lead to two derivative chromosomes. **(B)** Insertions result from a three break rearrangement and relocation of the chromosome segment from its original position. **(C)** Pericentric and **(D)** paracentric inversions are associated with two breakpoints on a single chromosome (arrowheads). In a pericentric inversion centromere is involved and break points in short and long arms occur. In paracentric inversion the centromere is not involved, and both breaks occur in the same arm. Balanced rearrangements may disrupt gene functions at the rearrangement breakpoints and cause chromosomally abnormal offspring, as well as recurrent miscarriages.

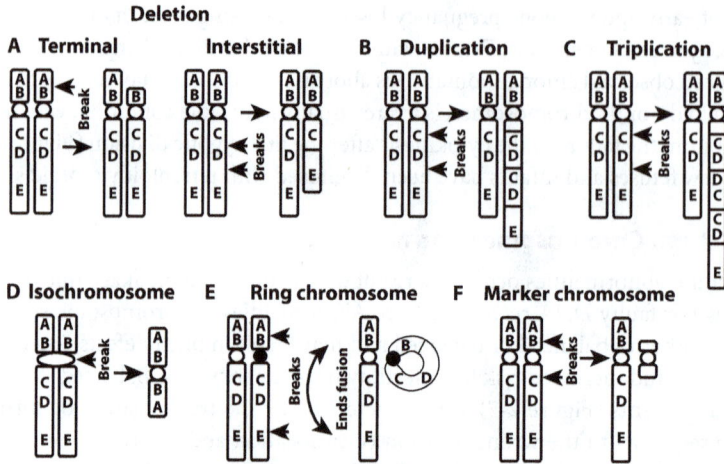

FIGURE 2-8. Schematic illustration of unbalanced structural chromosome rearrangements. (A) Terminal and interstitial deletions, and **(B)** duplication (two copies are present on the abnormal chromosome). Breaks occur in the DNA (arrowheads) followed by loss (deletion) or gain (duplication) of chromatin material between the breakpoints. **(C)** Triplication (three copies are present on the abnormal chromosome in addition to a one copy on the normal chromosome). Note that the middle copy is in an inverted orientation. **(D)** The isochromosome is composed of two copies of the same chromosome arm joined by a centromere. The isochromosome may replace one normal homologue or represent an extra chromosome. **(E)** A ring chromosome may result from the deletion of the distal portions of the short and long arms and fusion of the broken ends. Ring chromosomes also may be formed without detectable loss of genetic material. Ring chromosomes are unstable during division and may be lost or present in cells as multiple identical, or further rearranged copies. **(F)** A small marker chromosome composed of a centromere and pericentromeric regions. Marker chromosomes usually do not produce a recognizable G-banded pattern and can be visualized as extra chromosome on the karyotype.

Balanced Structural Rearrangements

A translocation is an abnormality in which chromosome segments are exchanged between two or more chromosomes (reciprocal translocation). In the general population, reciprocal translocations (Figure 2-7A) are relatively common, occurring in 1 out of 500 individuals. The vast majority of reciprocal translocations have unique breakpoints, making it difficult to predict the phenotype when it arises *de novo*. An exception is the translocation between the long arms of chromosome 11 and 22, t(11;22)(q23;q11.2), which always involves the same breakpoints. Carriers of t(11;22)(q23;q11.2) are at risk to have a child with an additional abnormal chromosome 22 composed of the proximal 22q and the distal 11q chromatin, also known as Emanuel syndrome.[14]

The Robertsonian translocation is a special form of rearrangement between two acrocentric chromosomes, resulting in the fusion of the long arms (Figure 2-9C). There are five pairs of acrocentric chromosomes (13, 14, 15, 21, and 22) characterized by very short arms (Figure 2-1). The short arms of acrocentric chromosomes are highly variable in size among healthy individuals, composed of noncoding repetitive satellite DNA, and therefore loss or gain of these regions is clinically benign. A Robertsonian translocation is the most frequent structural rearrangement in the general human population with frequency of approximately 1 in 1000. Carriers of Robertsonian translocations are at risk for chromosomally abnormal offspring, spontaneous abortions, and infertility.

Insertions, also known as balanced insertional translocations (Figure 2-7B), refer to the transposition of a chromosomal segment from its original location to a different location on the same chromosome or another nonhomologous chromosome. The incidence of insertions in the population is estimated to be 1 in 5000 people. In individuals with balanced insertions malsegregation during meiosis can result in the formation of unbalanced rearrangements, with either deletion (partial monosomy) or duplication (partial trisomy) of the insertion segment.

An inversion is a condition in which a chromosomal segment is present on the correct chromosome, but flipped 180 degree from its normal orientation (Figure 2-7C, D). Depending on the location of breakpoints, inversions are classified as pericentric, when the inverted segment includes the centromere (Figure 2-7C), or paracentric, when the centromere is excluded (Figure 2-7D). In general, inversions are found in approximately 1 out 7000 individuals. In meiosis, pairing of inverted segments are achieved by the formation of a loop, and based on the size of the inverted segment and number of crossovers within the loop, gametes may contain normal, inverted, or unbalanced chromosomes.

Balanced rearrangements usually are not associated with an abnormal phenotype, unless breakpoints disrupt dosage sensitive genes or DNA regulatory elements. However, carriers of balanced rearrangements are at increased risk for infertility, miscarriage, and abnormal progeny.[15] Balanced chromosome rearrangements are encountered among 1% to 2% of infertile individuals. Carriers of balanced abnormalities are often diagnosed following the birth of a child or miscarriage with unbalanced chromosome rearrangement. Parents of such children should undergo karyotype analysis to determine if one of the parents is a carrier for balanced chromosomal rearrangement. Carriers of balanced rearrangements have a theoretical risk of 50% to produce genetically unbalanced gametes. However, the actual risk of having a child with chromosomal abnormality and miscarriage is much less due to meiotic checkpoints that eliminate abnormal gametes, and actual risk will depend on the sex of the carrier (males are less likely to ejaculate sperm with abnormal karyotype due to more stringent meiotic checkpoint), type of chromosome, type of rearrangement, mode of segregation, size and orientation of the chromosome segments, and the number and location of breakpoints.

Unbalanced Structural Rearrangements

Unbalanced structural rearrangements are characterized by loss or gain of chromosomal DNA segments as a result of the rearrangement. Unbalanced structural

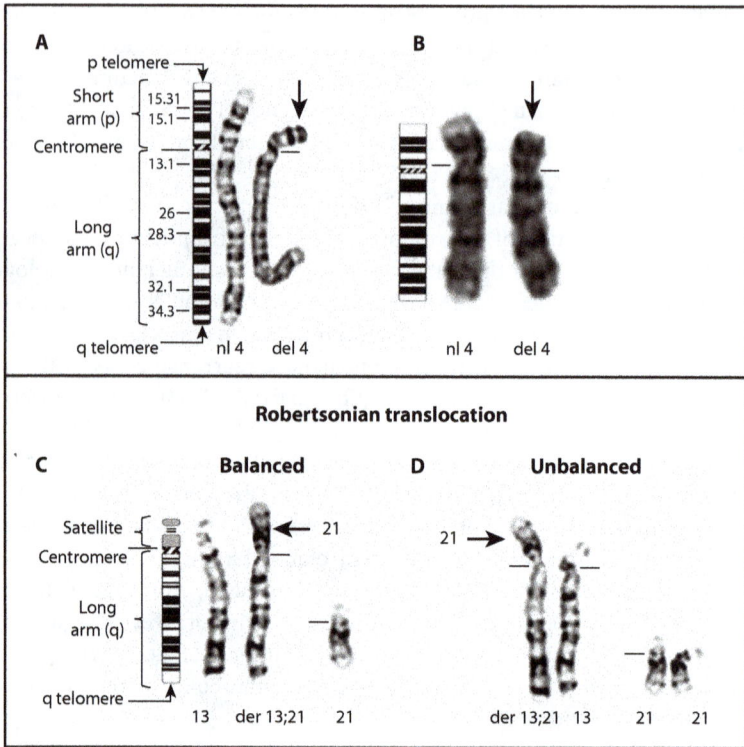

FIGURE 2-9. G-banded chromosomes with structural abnormalities. (A) A human chromosome 4 and its schematic representation (ideogram). Ideograms shows the relative size of the chromosome, its banding pattern, and centromere position. Two homologues are shown at 850 band resolution: a normal chromosome 4 (on the left) and an abnormal chromosome 4 (on the right) with a deletion in the short arm (arrow). This terminal deletion removes a segment involving 4p15.31-p16.3 bands and causes Wolf–Hirschhorn syndrome. **(B)** The chromosome 4 homologues and ideogram at 400 band resolution, obtained from the same patient with a terminal 4p deletion. **(C)** Balanced Robertsonian translocation between chromosome 13 and 21 in a parent. Carriers of a balanced Robertsonian translocation have 45 chromosomes, are phenotypically normal, but are at risk to pass the abnormal chromosome (13;21) to an offspring. **(D)** Partial karyotype of a child who inherited der(13;21) and a normal 21 from a carrier parent and normal chromosomes 13 and 21 from the another parent. A total three copies of chromosome 21 are present in the genome of this child, resulting in Down syndrome.

rearrangements include deletions (Figures 2-8A and 2-9A), duplications (Figure 2-8B), triplications (Figure 2-8C), the formation of isochromosomes (Figure 2-8D), ring chromosomes (Figure 2-8E), small chromosomes with an unidentifiable banding pattern, called marker chromosomes (Figure 2-8F), derivative chromosomes due to *de novo* unbalanced translocations or inherited from a balanced carrier parent, and complex chromosomal rearrangements. In contrast to numerical abnormalities that are greatly influenced by the age of the mother at the time of conception, the structural chromosome abnormalities can occur at any age and cannot be predicted.

Unbalanced structural rearrangements are generally associated with birth defects, developmental delay and/or intellectual impairment. However, some chromosomal rearrangements may have no effect on a person's health, particularly when the rearrangement involves a gene-poor region. Classic karyotype studies can only detect abnormalities larger than 5 to 10 Mb (megabase, million base pairs) in size. The human genome contains roughly 12 to 15 genes per 1 Mb, which means that roughly 60 to 150 genes need to be deleted or duplicated before the diagnosis can be made by these older techniques. Some genes are dosage sensitive, which means that the lack of one copy is detrimental and cannot be compensated by the presence of a second, presumably functioning copy. Losses and gains of dosage-sensitive genes can cause structural birth defects, mental retardation and syndromes. Because many of the adjacent genes are unrelated to each other, and are important, such losses can cause complex phenotypes. Losses and gains of such large segments will (1) decrease or increase the number of gene copies in the cell, and therefore influence protein levels and cell function; (2) remove or add gene regulatory elements that can affect genes outside of the deletion and/or duplication; (3) unmask mutation(s) that may exist on the second chromosome and cause a recessive disorder. The advent of molecular cytogenomics allows much better resolution and significantly improves detection of submicroscopic (smaller than 5 Mb) deletions and duplications.

Mosaicism

Constitutional mosaicism (true mosaicism) refers to condition when both genetically abnormal and normal diploid cells are present in various tissues of a body (somatic mosaicism), exist within one particular type of tissue (tissue specific mosaicism), or are found in the gonads (gonadal mosaicism). Approximately 50% of individuals with gonadal mosaicism also have mosaicism in other tissues, indicating that genetic events leading to mosaicism usually occur during early embryo development. Diagnosis of mosaicism is important for several reasons: the clinical phenotype may be significantly attenuated due to mosaicism and might be difficult to recognize; it may lead to cancer predisposition; and gonadal mosaicism may increase recurrence risk for a genetic condition in a family.

After fertilization, the zygote undergoes multiple mitotic divisions to give rise to the embryo and extraembryonic tissues (placenta). Nondisjunction during a postzygotic division may cause mosaicism in the placenta, fetus, or both (Figure 2-10). Indeed, more than 50% of cells within the preimplantation embryos show some degree of mosaicism.[16,17] Embryos with abnormal lines are either lost and do not implant, or the abnormal cell line within the embryo confers a growth disadvantage to the cell and is eliminated, or the abnormal cell line continues to replicate in the placenta. Confined placental mosaicism refers to the situation when a chromosome abnormality is only present in the placenta, but not in the fetus (Figure 2-10A).

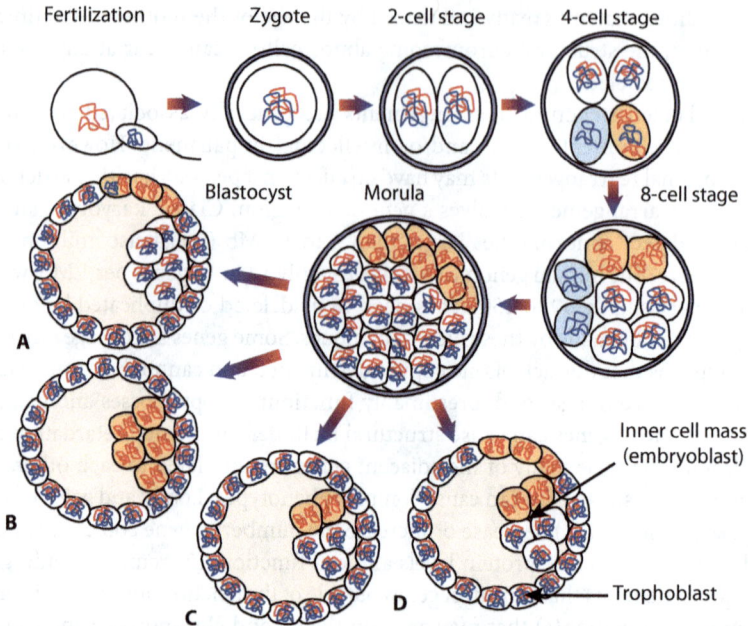

FIGURE 2-10. Origin of fetal mosaicism. Mitotic error at the four cell stage leads to trisomic (shaded orange) and monosomic (shaded blue) cell. At the eight-cell stage embryo, the cell with monosomy is eliminated and not present in the morula stage embryo. The trisomic cell (orange) loses the paternally inherited chromosome set and has maternal uniparental disomy for the remaining chromosome. If the affected chromosome is one of the known imprinted chromosomes (6, 7, 11, 14, and 15), then abnormal gene expression may lead to pathology (Table 2-1). The abnormal cell line may lead to mosaicism in the trophoblast (**A**), full uniparental disomy of the embryo (**B**), mosaic for uniparental disomy (**C**), and mosaic in both the trophoblast and embryo for uniparental disomy (**D**). Chorionic villus sampling combined with amniocentesis can help determine whether mosaicism is confined to the placenta, fetus or present in both.

Chromosomal mosaicism is detected in up to 2% of CVS, and in most cases it is confined to the placenta.[18] Confined placental mosaicism involving imprinted chromosomes, 6, 7, 11, 14, and 15 may indicate the presence of UPD in the corresponding fetus. Amniocentesis should be offered in such cases to rule out UPD. Finding an abnormal and normal cell population in CVS or amniotic fluid samples requires determination whether the abnormal cell line is the result of culture artifact (pseudomosaicism) or true mosaicism. Pseudomosaicism is likely when the abnormality is present in a single colony involving one or multiple cells, whereas true mosaicism is likely when abnormal cells are found in two or more independent primary cultures. Pseudomosaicism is found in 0.7% to 2.8% of amniotic fluid specimens, while the incidence of true mosaicism is much lower and observed in approximately 0.1% to 0.25% of cases.[19] True mosaicism is more likely to be associated with abnormal phenotype than pseudomosaicism.

Chimerism

Individuals with two distinct cell lines are usually diagnosed with mosaicism. However, when these cell lines show sex chromosome discrepancy, such as 46,XX and 46,XY karyotype, the findings may indicate chimerism.

Chimerism is a condition in which a fusion of two genetically different zygotes gives rise to a single embryo.[20] However, sex chromosome discrepancies, such as 46,XX/46,XY, are more commonly mosaicism that results from a postzygotic mitotic error in a single zygote, such as those with a 47,XXY or 46,XY chromosome constitution. True chimerism can be limited to hematopoietic cell lineage in the case of allogeneic stem cell transplantation or blood product transfusion, or it can arise from transplacental cell exchange between twins or between a mother and her fetus. True chimerism is a rare condition in individuals with heterosexual 46,XX/46,XY chromosome composition and ambiguous genitalia. Same sex chimerism does exist, but has not been associated with health problems.

REFERENCES

1. Armanios M, Blackburn EH. The telomere syndromes. Nature reviews. *Genetics.* 2012;13:693-704.

2. Wilcox AJ, Weinberg CR, O'Connor JF, et al. Incidence of early loss of pregnancy. *N Engl J Med.* 1988;319:189-194.

3. Wilcox AJ, Baird DD, Weinberg CR. Time of implantation of the conceptus and loss of pregnancy. *N Engl J Med.* 1999;340:1796-1799.

4. Delhanty JD. Inherited aneuploidy: germline mosaicism. *Cytogenet Genome Res.* 2011;133:136-140.

5. Warburton D, Dallaire L, Thangavelu M, et al. Trisomy recurrence: a reconsideration based on North American data. *Am J Hum Genet.* 2004;75:376-385.

6. Yamazawa K, Ogata T, Ferguson-Smith AC. Uniparental disomy and human disease: an overview. *Am J Med Genet. Part C, Seminars in Medical Genetics.* 2012;154C:329-334.

7. Liehr T. Cytogenetic contribution to uniparental disomy (UPD). *Mol Cytogenet.* 2012;3:8.

8. Feuk L, Carson AR, Scherer SW. Structural variation in the human genome. *Nat Rev Genet.* 2006;7:85-97.

9. Lupski JR. Genomic rearrangements and sporadic disease. *Nat Genet.* 2007;39;S43-47.

10. Hassold T, Hall H, Hunt P. The origin of human aneuploidy: where we have been, where we are going. *Hum Mol Genet.* 2007;16 Spec No. 2:R203-208.

11. Hassold T, Hunt P. To err (meiotically) is human: the genesis of human aneuploidy. *Nat Rev Genet.* 2001;2:280-291.

12. Mori MA, Lapunzina P, Delicado A, et al. A prenatally diagnosed patient with full monosomy 21: ultrasound, cytogenetic, clinical, molecular, and necropsy findings. *Am J Med Genet.* 2004;127A:69-73.

13. Sybert VP, McCauley E. Turner's syndrome. *N Engl J Med.* 2004;351:1227-1238.

14. Carter MT, St Pierre SA, Zackai EH. Phenotypic delineation of Emanuel syndrome (supernumerary derivative 22 syndrome): clinical features of 63 individuals. *Am J Med Genet.* 2009;149A:1712-1721.

15. Bugge M, Bruun-Petersen G, Brondum-Nielsen K, et al. Disease associated balanced chromosome rearrangements: a resource for large scale genotype-phenotype delineation in man. *J Med Genet.* 2000;37:858-865.

16. Santos MA, Teklenburg G, Macklon NS, et al. The fate of the mosaic embryo: chromosomal constitution and development of Day 4, 5 and 8 human embryos. *Hum Reprod.* 2010;25:1916-1926.

17. Vanneste E, Voet T, Le Caignec C, et al. Chromosome instability is common in human cleavage-stage embryos. *Nat Med.* 2009;15:577-583.

18. Hahnemann JM, Vejerslev LO. European collaborative research on mosaicism in CVS (EUCROMIC)—fetal and extrafetal cell lineages in 192 gestations with CVS mosaicism involving single autosomal trisomy. *Am J Med Genet.* 1997;70:179-187.

19. Hsu LY, Kaffe S, Jenkins EC, et al. Proposed guidelines for diagnosis of chromosome mosaicism in amniocytes based on data derived from chromosome mosaicism and pseudomosaicism studies. *Prenat Diagn.* 1992;12:555-573.

20. Malan V, Vekemans M, Turleau C. Chimera and other fertilization errors. *Clin Genet.* 2006;70:363-373.

Patterns of Inheritance

■ PRINCIPLES OF MENDELIAN INHERITANCE

Mendelian disorders result from a mutation at a single genetic locus. A locus may be present on an autosome or on a sex chromosomes, and it may manifest in a dominant or a recessive mode. There are over 10,000 traits believed to be inherited in a mendelian fashion, but only a few of the more common disorders of interest to the obstetrician-gynecologist have been highlighted in this chapter to illustrate patterns of inheritance.

The patterns of inheritance for the various mendelian traits are illustrated by the idealized pedigrees in Figure 3-1. An autosomal recessive trait (disease) is expressed only when the mutant gene is present in a double dose (homozygous state). Both parents are heterozygous and possess one copy of the mutant gene and one copy of the normal or functional gene. Autosomal recessive traits are characterized as follows:

1. There is rarely a positive family history outside the affected sibship.
2. Males and females are equally likely to be affected.
3. Heterozygous parents are usually unaffected and have a 25% chance of producing an offspring affected with the disease.

Autosomal dominant traits manifest in the heterozygous state (single-gene dose) and are characterized by the following:

1. They can be transmitted from generation to generation.
2. The probability that a person carrying the gene will pass it on to his or her offspring is 50%.
3. Males and females are equally likely to be affected.

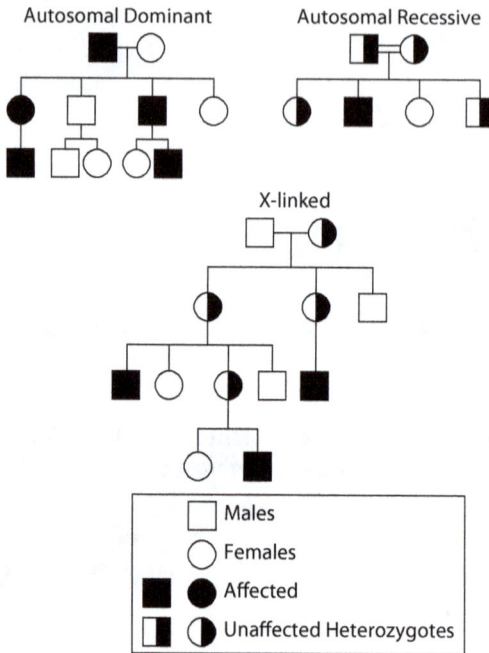

FIGURE 3-1. Idealized pedigree illustrating patterns of mendelian inheritance.

Males (XY) and females (XX) differ in the number of X chromosomes they possess. As a result, the inheritance pattern of mutations carried on the X-chromosome will differ from the inheritance pattern of mutations on autosomes. A recessive trait controlled by a gene on the X chromosome will be expressed in all males carrying the allele. Affected males are said to be hemizygous. Females will be affected if they are homozygous or if they inactivate most of the X chromosomes carrying the normal allele. The following are characteristics of X-linked inheritance:

1. There is no male-to-male transmission.
2. All daughters of an affected male receive the mutant gene and are therefore carriers.
3. One-half of the sons, and one-half of the daughters of a heterozygous female receive the mutant gene.

The distinction between X-linked dominant and X-linked recessive is unclear, but in general, *X-linked recessive* refers to a trait that is not clinically expressed in the heterozygous female, and *X-linked dominant* to a trait that is expressed in the heterozygous female.

Case 1: Ms. Carey is a 25-year-old who presents for her first prenatal visit at 10 weeks' gestation. Her medical history is negative but she gives a history that her 35-year-old sister has myotonic dystrophy. Her parents are in their mid-60s, and have no significant health problems. Her husband's family history is negative for any issues that would place her pregnancy at risk.

Neurologic Diseases. The onset of many of the autosomal dominant neurologic diseases occurs in adulthood, and these diseases are generally more familiar to the neurologist than to the obstetrician-gynecologist. However, two of these disorders—myotonic dystrophy and Huntington disease—will be discussed to illustrate the necessity of having a basic knowledge of the mechanisms of inheritance and the clinical implications of these disorders.

Myotonic dystrophy (MD) is a condition characterized by myotonia, cataracts, and other variable features, such as male-pattern baldness.[1] The onset of symptoms usually occurs in the third or fourth decade of life. In addition to the adult form, there is neonatal form of the disorder, known as *congenital myotonic dystrophy*. This disorder is characterized by severe hypotonia, respiratory compromise, and often death in the newborn period. Those infants who do survive commonly have severe developmental delay.

The MD gene is characterized by a repeated sequence of cytosine-thymidine-guanine (CTG), which in normal persons is repeated between 5 and 34 times. This "trinucleotide repeat" is expanded to greater than 100 repeats in persons affected with adult-onset MD. Neonates with congenital MD may have more than 2000 copies of the repeat. Figure 3-2 presents a pedigree of a family that represents Case 1. The patient (proband) presents at 10 weeks' gestation with a history that her sister has adult-onset MD. Neither of her parents, both in their mid-60s have

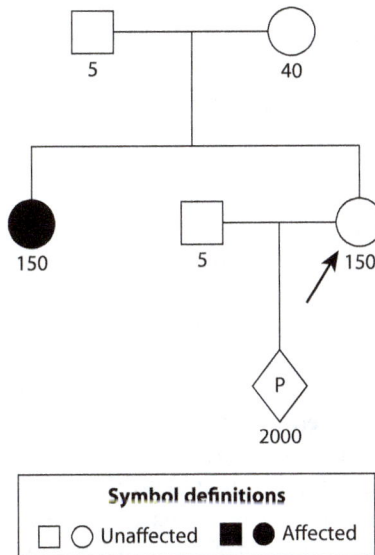

FIGURE 3-2. Pedigree of a family with an apparently isolated case of myotonic dystrophy (shaded circle). Molecular studies for trinucleotide repeats are depicted under each symbol. The number of repeats in the proband (arrow) is similar to that of her affected sister, and the proband can be expected to experience symptoms in the future. Her fetus has 2000 repeats, consistent with the diagnosis of congenital myotonic dystrophy. Her mother has a premutation (40 repeats).

any symptoms to suggest that either is affected with MD. Based on the absence of any symptoms in the patient or her parents, we might assume that the sister's disease represents a new dominant mutation. Molecular testing of the family, however, indicates a much different scenario:

- The sister has 150 trinucleotide repeats, consistent with her clinical symptoms.
- Her mother has 40 repeats, which is in the range of what is called a *premutation* (35-100 repeats).
- The proband also has 150 repeats and can be expected to experience MD symptoms in the future.
- Molecular evaluation reveals that the fetus has 2000 repeats, consistent with the diagnosis of congenital MD.

Trinucleotide repeat disorders are characterized by the presence of unstable premutations that may remain unchanged or may amplify during spermatogenesis or oogenesis. In the case of MD, marked amplification can occur when the gene is passed from the mother, but not from the father. Therefore, the congenital form of MD is seen only when the gene is passed from the mother to the fetus. Determination of the status of a person with a family history of MD (ie, normal, premutation, full mutation) is quite precise with the use of modern molecular techniques.

Huntington disease (HD) is a late-onset, progressive, and fatal disease, inherited in a classic autosomal-dominant fashion. The early symptoms of the disease are subtle loss of muscle coordination, forgetfulness, and personality changes. The disease progresses in stages, from choreiform movements (hence the older name of Huntington chorea) to hypokinesis and then to rigidity. Ultimately, the patient is bedridden with dysphagia, dysarthria, and impairment of gait and coordination. Onset of the disease occurs most commonly between the ages of 30 and 50 years.

Like MD, HD has been found to be caused by a mutation involving a trinucleotide repeat sequence. Normal persons have between 11 and 31 copies of a CAG repeat. The full mutation range is between 38 and 100 copies. There is an intermediate range of 32 to 38 repeats, and there are examples of both affected and unaffected persons with this number of repeats.[2] Therefore, there does not appear to be a true premutation in HD. Unlike MD, inheritance of HD from the father is associated with expansion of the repeats and an earlier age of onset. In approximately one-third of cases where the father passes on the gene to his offspring, there is an expansion resulting in juvenile-onset HD.

The ability to diagnose HD precisely by molecular techniques offers both the possibility of presymptomatic (predictive) testing and prenatal detection of an affected fetus. Although predictive testing can offer freedom from the psychological burdens associated with being at risk if the person does not carry the mutation, the impact on persons found to have the gene can be devastating. Those found to carry the gene face the inevitability of developing a disease for which there is currently no treatment.

Most commonly the obstetrician-gynecologist will be presented with the request for prenatal testing by an at-risk patient. It must be emphasized to the couple that testing will determine precisely whether the fetus has the HD gene.

Thus, a positive result gives an at-risk patient a presymptomatic diagnosis of HD. Direct prenatal testing should not be performed unless an at-risk patient has already undergone predictive testing. One option to avoid the difficulties of direct prenatal testing is the use of preimplantation genetic diagnosis, which only provides information regarding unaffected embryos, and does not reveal the status of the at-risk parent.[3,4]

Because of the significant ethical, psychological, and medical issues associated with predictive testing, such testing should take place only at institutions where protocols are in place for pre- and post-testing counseling and support.[5]

Autosomal Dominant Conditions of Interest to the OB/GYN

Skeletal Dysplasias. Until recently, the diagnosis of skeletal dysplasia in children was dependent on radiographic and physical features. Because of the often subtle variations between categories and the limitations of ultrasonography, prenatal detection was limited only to the most severe types. With the discovery of the molecular basis for many of these conditions, a precise prenatal diagnosis can now be determined as early as the first trimester via chorionic villus sampling (CVS), and in some cases by noninvasive prenatal testing (NIPT) on a maternal blood sample.[6,7]

Achondroplasia. Achondroplasia is the single most common skeletal dysplasia in humans. Inherited in an autosomal-dominant fashion, a person with achondroplasia has a 50% chance of having a child with the disorder. Because the gene is 100% penetrant, a person will have the disease if the gene is inherited. The discovery that achondroplasia results from a mutation in a gene known as fibroblast growth factor receptor 3 (FGFR-3) now enables a precise diagnosis in subsequent pregnancies, either by amniocentesis or CVS, or NIPT.[8]

FGFR-3 mutations also have been found to cause a lethal dwarfism known as *thanatophoric dysplasia*. It represents a new dominant mutation with an empiric risk of recurrence of approximately 5% (see discussion of germ cell mosaicism in Chapter 2). Molecular testing can be done to confirm the diagnosis in cases where severe short-limb dwarfism is diagnosed on the basis of ultrasound examination. Using amniotic fluid cells, one can make a precise diagnosis and therefore provide the family with more exact prognostic information.

Osteogenesis Imperfecta. Osteogenesis imperfecta (OI) describes a constellation of disorders characterized by brittle bones and defects in type I collagen. The form of OI of significance for the obstetrician-gynecologist is the perinatal lethal form, OI type II. Also, a new dominant mutation in most circumstances, it can most easily be diagnosed by assays of collagen structure.[9] If these assays are performed on fibroblasts from the affected child, prenatal diagnosis is straightforward in any subsequent pregnancy. There is, however, one major caveat: because this analysis is of protein structure, not DNA sequence, future pregnancies must be evaluated by CVS, not amniocentesis. Collagen defects can be analyzed in chorionic villi, but not in aminocytes. A second caveat is the necessity to fully evaluate the index case with both biochemical and molecular based studies. Some forms of lethal osteogenesis may be the result of recessive inheritance, not new dominant mutations. In these cases both parents carry a mutant gene and the risk for recurrence is 25%. In these cases DNA based studies would be offered in subsequent pregnancies.[10,11]

> **Case 2:** Ms. Jeune is a 20-year-old at 6 weeks' gestation in her first pregnancy. Her past medical history is entirely unremarkable. In taking her family history, she gives you a history that her only sibling, a male, died at age 2 of what she described as "undeveloped lungs." She also was told by her parents that her brother had a "problem with how his bones developed." How would you manage this pregnancy?

In Case 2 the family history is quite suggestive of a skeletal dysplasia that was associated with a small chest, and pulmonary hypoplasia, ultimately leading to early death. The fact that the child lived for 2 years makes one of the severe "lethal" disorders, such as thanatophoric dysplasia unlikely. Every attempt should be made to get medical records on the child, which hopefully include a specific diagnosis, and if not, laboratory testing, imaging, or an autopsy that could assist a geneticist in making a presumptive diagnosis. Records were obtained on this patient and confirmed the presence of a skeletal dysplasia. The precise diagnosis was Jeune thoracic dystrophy. It is inherited in an autosomal recessive fashion. In counseling this patient a key precept of AR inheritance must be remembered. Both of our patient's parents must be carriers of the mutated gene. Therefore, they have a one-fourth chance of an affected child, a one-half chance of having children who are carriers, and a one-fourth chance of a child with two normal genes. In a theoretical family of four, there would be one affected, two carriers, and one who did not inherit the gene in question. For our patient who does not have the disease, there are only three possible genotypes, two of which are carriers. Therefore, like all siblings of individuals with recessive diseases, she has a two-third chance of carrying the gene. Because of the rarity of the condition, her spouse is unlikely to carry the gene mutations, but referral of the couple to a geneticist is appropriate to discuss testing options.

Autosomal Recessive Disorders of Interest to the OB/GYN

Among the autosomal recessive diseases, the hemoglobinopathies play a significant role in Ob/Gyn. Hemoglobin is a tetrameric protein consisting of four globin chains. In humans, there are six structurally different types of globin chains: alpha (α), beta (β), gamma (γ), delta (δ), epsilon (ε), and zeta (ζ). The synthesis of various chains is switched on and off during the process of differentiation and may represent an adaptive process for the developing fetus. The embryonic chains (ε and ζ) are rapidly replaced as the fetus develops. Each of the different hemoglobins found in humans is formed by the combination of two α-chains and two non-α-chains (γ, β, δ).[12]

The messenger RNA (mRNA) for each globin gene is transcribed from a varying number of genes, which may differ among populations. It appears that, in general, there are four genes controlling α-chain synthesis and two controlling β-chain synthesis. Genes for the α-chains are located on chromosome 16, and those for β, γ, and δ are located on chromosome 11. In the hemoglobinopathies, the specific disorder may be considered recessive, because heterozygous persons have half the genes (either one or two) functioning to make the normal protein and half functioning to making no protein or an abnormal one. Therefore, either the homozygous state or a double heterozygous state (ie, two different deleterious mutations) can result in a hemoglobinopathy.

α-*Thalassemia* is characterized by a deficiency in α-globin chain synthesis. Normal α-chain production is the product of four functioning α genes (two on each chromosome 16). Therefore, either one or both genes can be deleted on a chromosome 16, resulting in four clinical states according to the number of functional α-globin genes (3, 2, 1, or 0). Of clinical significance is the circumstance in which there is one functional gene, known as hemoglobin H disease, or 0 functional genes, known as hemoglobin Barts disease, which results in fetal hydrops.

Of importance to the obstetrician-gynecologist is the clinical presentation of the homozygous form of the disorder. The mother usually presents with severe preeclampsia in the early third trimester, and ultrasound evaluation reveals hydrops fetalis. Because of the lethal nature of this condition and the significant maternal morbidity, all patients of Asian ancestry should be screened for the carrier state of α-thalassemia. A simple screening tool is a complete blood count with red cell indices. Carriers of the α-thalassemia mutation have a mild anemia and a mean corpuscular volume of less than 80 femtoliters (fl). Currently, the simplest method for the diagnosis of α-thalassemia carriers is to exclude iron deficiency anemia by appropriate studies, and to exclude the carrier state for β-thalassemia by hemoglobin electrophoresis. Because both parents must be carriers in order to have an affected fetus, the next step at this point should be to test the woman's partner. If he also appears to be a carrier, appropriate molecular studies can be done to confirm the diagnosis in both parents. When both parents are confirmed to be carriers, prenatal diagnosis is possible either by CVS or amniocentesis.

β-*Thalassemia* is defined as either reduced (β+) or absent (βo) β-chain synthesis. β-thalassemia is prevalent in areas of the world where malaria is endemic (Mediterranean area, Africa, Middle East, India, Southeast Asia, and Southern China). Based on knowledge of the mutations that are specific to a geographic region or ethnic group, one can use a PCR-based screening protocol to detect approximately 80% of the common mutations, and many of the rare mutations.

As with α-thalassemia, the simplest initial approach to screening for β-thalassemia is to obtain a complete blood count with red cells indices. When the mean corpuscular volume is less than 80 fl, hemoglobin electrophoresis is indicated. Carriers of the β-thalassemia gene will have an elevated level of hemoglobin A_2 (>3.5% of total hemoglobin will be A_2). If the partner is also found to be a carrier, appropriate molecular studies must then be performed to determine the exact mutations before prenatal diagnosis can be offered.[13]

Case 3: Ms. Lubs presents for a preconception visit with you. Her medical and surgical history is negative. She gives a family history that her paternal uncle has mental retardation. No other family members have

intellectual or learning disabilities. She is concerned that she will have a child with mental retardation. How would you counsel her?

Fragile-X Syndrome. Fragile-X syndrome is the most common inherited form of mental retardation, affecting approximately 1 in 2500 men and 1 in 4000 women.[14] Therefore approximately 1 in 200 women in the general population may be carriers of the gene. Fragile-X syndrome has a wide range of clinical presentations, including moderate disabilities in females, autism, and other psychiatric disorders.

Unlike classic X-linked disorders (eg, DMD, hemophilia), fragile-X syndrome affects both males and females; it is important to note that there are males who carry the gene, but have normal intelligence and no physical stigmata of the disorder. This variable clinical phenotype reflects the novel mutation in the gene known as fragile-X mental retardation 1 (*FMR1*). The *FMR1* gene is characterized by a repeated sequence of the trinucleotide cytosine-guanine-guanine (CGG) in the 5′ untranslated region of gene. In unaffected persons, between 5 and 44 repeats of this sequence are found. Intellectually normal carriers of the mutation have between 56 and 200 CGG repeats, called a premutation. In carrier females, premutations are unstable and may undergo further expansion during oogenesis. If the CGG sequence expands beyond 200 repeats, it is considered a full mutation, and all males with this number of repeats will show the clinical features of fragile-X syndrome, and approximately one-half of females likewise will have mental retardation. Males with the premutation do not have expansion during spermatogenesis, but will pass the premutation to all of their daughters, each of which will be at risk for having an affected child.

Table 3-1 outlines clinical situations that should prompt screening for fragile-X syndrome, either in a pregnant patient or in the patient presenting for preconception counseling. Two of these recommendations are straightforward, but the latter two require explanation. We traditionally have assumed that X-linked disorders in the patient's father's family (paternal side) would not place the pregnancy at risk. In the case of fragile-X syndrome, however, the gene is nonpenetrant in 20% of males with the fragile-X gene (ie, they do not show clinical symptoms). Therefore, a patient's father who has a family history of mental retardation may carry the fragile-X premutation, which he will pass to all of his daughters. In the circumstance where the patient's paternal uncle has unexplained mental retardation (Case 3), her risk of being a carrier of the fragile-X gene is approximately 1 in 100.

■ TABLE 3-1. Indications for Fragile-X Screening

- Family history of known Fragile-X related disorders.
- Family history of unexplained mental retardation or developmental delay.
- Family history of autism.
- Family history of premature ovarian sufficiency.
- Personal history of premature ovarian insufficiency or an elevated follicle-stimulating hormone (FSH) level before the age of 40.

Therefore, any history of unexplained mental retardation should prompt testing for fragile-X carrier status.

Of particular interest to the obstetrician-gynecologist is the association of fragile-X premutation and premature ovarian insufficiency. Testing for FMRI mutations in circumstances where there is a family history of premature menopause is indicated (see Chapter 14 for further discussion).

> **Case 4: Ms. Simpson is a 20-year-old primigravida who presents at 12 weeks' gestation. Her medical and family history is negative, but her husband was diagnosed at birth with a sacral spina bifida. Repair was done immediately after birth, and he has no residual neurological defects. She would like to know whether her pregnancy is at risk for being affected with spina bifida.**

■ MULTIFACTORIAL/POLYGENIC INHERITANCE

There are many genetic conditions that recur in families much more commonly than would be expected by chance alone. There also are many adult-onset disease that seem to "run in families," and have a genetic predisposition. The terms "multifactorial" and "polygenic" have been used to describe these conditions. In the past, the explanation has been that a combination of genes with, or without, environmental factors results in a specific condition. The classic examples for this "multifactorial" inheritance are the neural tube defects (anencephaly, encephalocele, and spina bifida). Although the incidence of neural tube defects (NTD) in the general population is only 1 to 2 per 1000 livebirths, the risk of recurrence following the birth of an affected child is 2% to 3%. Unlike mendelian traits, the risk of recurrence increases with each subsequent affected child, increasing to 5% to 10% after two affected children. In the case of NTD one of the known environmental determinants is dietary folate. Increasing intake of folic acid prior to a subsequent pregnancy and throughout the period of organogenesis has been shown to reduce the risk of recurrence by nearly 75%.

Genetic disorders that are inherited in a multifactorial fashion have certain consistent characteristics:

- The disorder usually involves a single organ system, or organs that develop together embryologically.
- Unlike mendelian disorders, the risk of recurrence increases following each affected pregnancy.
- The more serious the malformation, the higher the risk of recurrence. For example, a bilateral cleft lip/cleft palate increases the risk of recurrence greater than an unilateral cleft lip/cleft palate.
- If a particular malformation is known to occur more frequently among members of one sex, then the risk for recurrence is higher in a family where the index case is of the less frequently affected sex. For example, pyloric stenosis occurs more frequently in males. Therefore, the recurrence risk will be higher in a family with a daughter who has pyloric stenosis.

Many of the common birth defects are inherited in a multifactorial fashion, and include NTD, congenital heart defects, cleft lip and/or palate, and club feet. As the specific genes are determined that are causative for these malformations, and the key environmental influences are elicited, a more precise understanding of the inheritance will be developed. With that greater understanding, hopefully a more precise term will be put forward to explain this "multifactorial/polygenic" inheritance.

Our patient in Case 4 has a 2% to 3% risk that her fetus will have a NTD. The risk to the fetus is the same for both an affected parent, or an affected sibling, as both are first degree relatives. Had she presented prior to conception she would have been a candidate for 4 mg of folate daily. By 10 weeks' gestation no benefit would be gained by recommending the increased dosage of folic acid. It is important to counsel the patient that the type and severity of a potential NTD is not directly related to the defect her husband had. In this pregnancy, the patient should be offered maternal serum α-fetoprotein testing and a detailed ultrasound at 18 weeks' gestation. Alternatively, she could be offered amniocentesis at 16 weeks' to assess amniotic fluid α-fetoprotein. Prior to any subsequent pregnancy, she should be encouraged to take the 4 mg daily dosage of folic acid.

REFERENCES

1. Johnson NE, Heatwole CR. Myotonic dystrophy: from bench to bedside. *Semin Neurol*. 2012;32(3):246-254.

2. Huntington's Disease Collaborative Research Group. A novel gene containing a trinucleotide repeat that is unstable and expanded on Huntington's disease chromosomes. *Cell*. 1993;72:971-983.

3. Van Rij MC, De Rademaeker M, Moutou C, et al. Preimplantation genetic diagnosis (PGD) for Huntington's disease: the experience of three European centres. *Eur J Hum Genet*. 2012;20(4):368-375.

4. Erez A, Plunkett K, Sutton VR, McGuire AL. The right to ignore genetic risk in the genomic era-prenatal testing for Huntington disease as a paradigm. *Am J Med Genet*. 2010;7:1774-1780.

5. Dufrasne S, Roy M, Galvez, M, Rosenblatt DS. Experience over fifteen years with a protocol for predictive testing for Huntington disease. *Mol Genet Metab*. 2011;102(4):494-504.

6. Chitty LS, Griffin DR, Meaney C, et al. New aids for the non-invasive prenatal diagnosis of achondroplasia: dysmorphic features, charts of fetal size and molecular confirmation using cell-free fetal DNA in maternal plasma. *Ultrasound Obstet Gynecol*. 2011;37(3):283-289.

7. Chitty LS, Khalil A, Barrett AN, et al. Safe, accurate, prenatal diagnosis of thanatophoric dysplasia using ultrasound and free fetal DNA. *Prenat Diagn*. 2013;33(5):416-423.

8. Rousseau F, Bonaventure, J, Legeai-Mallet L, et al. Mutations in the gene encoding fibroblast growth factor receptor-3 in achondroplasia. *Nature*. 1994;371:252-254.

9. Pepin M, Atkinson M, Starman, BJ, Byers PH. Strategies and outcomes of prenatal diagnosis of osteogenesis imperfecta: a review of biochemical and molecular studies completed in 129 pregnancies. *Prenat Diagn*. 1997;17:559-570.

10. Pyott SM, Pepin MG, Schwarze U, et al. Recurrence of perinatal lethal osteogenesis imperfecta in sibships: parsing the risk between parental mosaicism for dominant mutations and autosomal recessive inheritance. *Genet Med.* 2011;13(2):125-130.

11. Van Dijk FS, Nesbitt IM, Nikkels PG, et al. CRTAP mutations in lethal and severe osteogenesis imperfecta: the importance of combining biochemical and molecular genetic analysis. *Eur J Hum Genet.* 2009;17(12):1560-1569.

12. Cao A, Kan YW. The prevention of thalassemia. *Cold Spring Harb Perspect Med.* 2013;3:a011775.

13. Tongson T, Charoenkwan P, Sirivatanapa P. Effectiveness of the model for prenatal control of severe thalassemia. *Prenat Diagn.* 2013;33(5):477-483.

14. Bagni C, Tassone F, Neri G, Hagerman R. Fragile X syndrome: causes, diagnosis, mechanism, and therapeutics. *J Clin Invest.* 2012;122:4314-4322.

Taking a Family History

Case 1: A 30-year-old G_3P_2 presents for her new OB visit at 10 weeks' gestation. She has had two full-term uncomplicated vaginal deliveries. Her second child, a boy now age 4, has recently been diagnosed with severe intellectual disability. Her family history is remarkable for a brother and two maternal uncles who have been diagnosed with "mental retardation."

A good family history is an important tool for making a diagnosis, and giving anticipatory guidance for many medical conditions, but is especially important for genetic conditions. The family history is essential for genetic counseling, including discussion of reproductive planning and understanding recurrence risks. Recording an accurate family history requires obtaining information on specific illnesses and medical conditions in family members, as well as pregnancy histories of female members. The importance of a family history is not to recognize a specific genetic disorder, but to uncover familial patterns of birth defects, cognitive disabilities, malignancies, or other medical problems. The information obtained may be important for early diagnosis, timely management and treatment, or reproductive planning. It should be updated at least annually, or sooner if new pertinent information is obtained.

■ CONSTRUCTING A PEDIGREE

Obtaining a family history can be time consuming, but the information obtained is invaluable for providing quality patient care.[1] Although the use of checklists may be helpful in identifying areas of concern, it may miss key information that can be obtained by more direct questioning about the health of closely related family members. The most helpful method for recording a family history is the pedigree, which allows the identification of patterns that give clues to a potentially inherited disorder. Genetic counselors construct at least a three generation pedigree using standard symbols (Figure 4-1). Females are designated by circles, males by squares, and miscarriages or stillbirths of unknown gender by diamonds. Some geneticists use triangles or small filled circles to represent miscarriages. A deceased individual is designated with a diagonal line drawn through the symbol. Ages of death or gestational ages of the pregnancy loss should be written under the appropriate symbol. Symbols of individuals affected with a disorder should have their symbol shaded in, and the designation as to what the shading indicates should be given on a key on the pedigree. By convention the proband (patient) is denoted by an arrow. In denoting relationships, the male is placed on the left, and the female on the right, connected by a horizontal line. As noted in Figure 4-1, children are placed below the parents connected by a vertical line, and in the order of birth. Miscarriages and other pregnancy losses should be included in the appropriate birth order. Figure 4-2 shows a three generation pedigree for our case example with mental retardation that affects only males, and is inherited through unaffected females, strongly suggestive of an X-linked recessive form of mental retardation. The key features are that (1) only males are affected, (2) there is no male to male transmission, and (3) the gene of interest appears to be passing through carrier females.

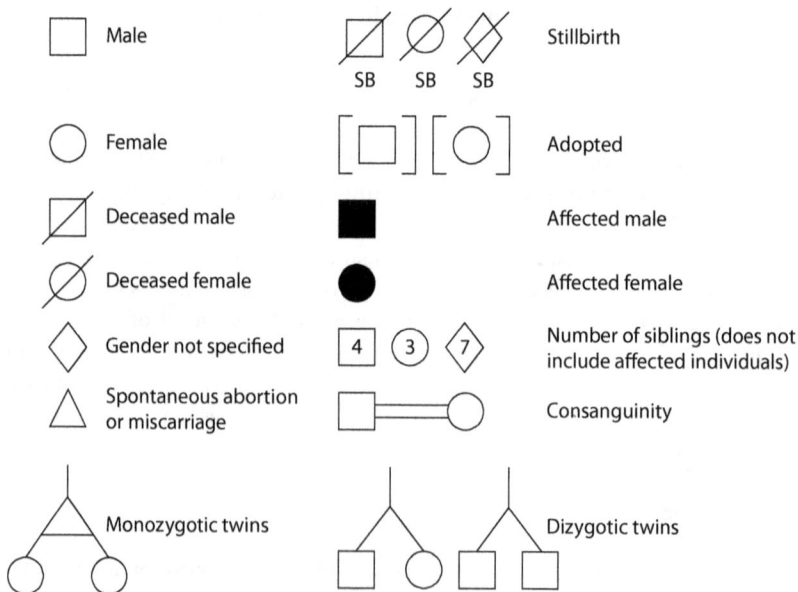

FIGURE 4-1. Standard symbols in a pedigree.

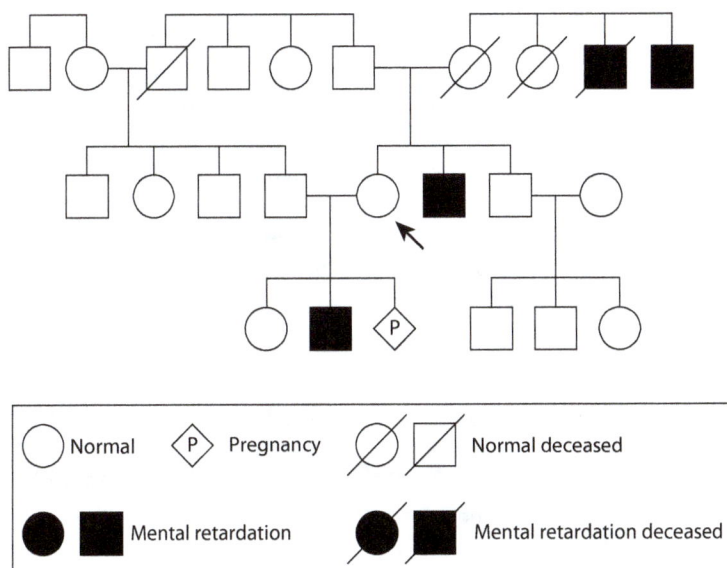

FIGURE 4-2. Pedigree of case 1.

■ KEY QUESTIONS TO ASK

There are six questions that are good starting points to getting to key genetic issues.[2] They are

1. Are there any health problems that are known to run in your family, or that close relatives have been told are genetic?
2. Is there anyone in the family who had cancer, heart disease, or other adult-onset medical conditions at an early age (between 20 and 50 years old)?
3. Does/did anyone in the family have intellectual disabilities, learning problems, or have to go to a special school?
4. Have there been early deaths in the family, including stillbirths, infant deaths, multiple miscarriages, or childhood deaths?
5. Has any relative had extreme or unexpected reactions to medications or anesthesia?
6. Have there been any problems with pregnancy, issues with infertility or birth defects in your family?

It is essential to use terminology that is understandable to the family. Although the medically correct term is "intellectual disability," the patient may think of the uncle as having "mental retardation" or as being "slow." Likewise, all bleeding disorders may be described as "hemophilia," even in women. When the pedigree suggests a potential risk to the patient or her offspring, obtaining medical records is essential to providing adequate genetic counseling.

■ ETHNIC AND RACIAL BACKGROUND IMPLICATIONS

As part of the pedigree, the racial and ethnic origins of the patient and her spouse should be noted. Certain geographic, ethnic, and racial groups are at relatively high risk for otherwise rare genetic disorders. The high frequency reflects both evolutionary forces, and geographic/cultural isolation. For example, sickle cell carriers of African ancestry seem to carry some protection from malaria. On the other hand, individuals of Ashkenazi Jewish ancestry are at risk for certain disorders, such as Tay-Sachs disease, because of a combination of geographic and cultural issues that are part of their heritage. Table 4-1 outlines diseases prevalent in certain racial/ethnic groups.[3]

■ **TABLE 4-1.** Examples of Genetic Disorders Seen in Specific Ethnic and Racial Groups

Racial or Ethnic Group	Genetic Disorder	Inheritance
African American	Sickle cell disease	AR
	Glucose-6-phosphate dehydrogenase deficiency	XLR
Amish/Mennonite	Maple syrup urine disease	AR
	Chondroectodermal dysplasia (Ellis-van Crevald syndrome)	AR
	Cartilage-hair hypoplasia	AR
	McKusick-Kaufman syndrome	AR
	Limb girdle muscular dystrophy	AR
	Glutaric Aciduria type I	AR
Ashkenazi Jewish	Tay-Sachs disease	AR
	Canavan disease	AR
	Gaucher disease type 1	AR
	Hereditary breast/ovarian cancer	AD
	Sensorineural deafness	AR
	Familial dysautonomia	AR
	Mucolipidosis type IV	AR
	Niemann-Pick disease type A	AR
Finnish	Hereditary nephrosis	AR
	Cartilage-hair hypoplasia	AR
	Infantile neuronal ceroid lipofuscinosis	AR
French Canadian	Leigh syndrome, French-Canadian type	AR
	Hereditary multiple intestinal atresia	AR
	Tyrosinemia type I	AR
	Tay-Sachs disease	AR
	Cystinosis	AR
	Pseudo-vitamin D-deficiency rickets	AR

(Continued)

■ **TABLE 4-1.** Examples of Genetic Disorders Seen in Specific Ethnic and Racial Groups (*Continued*)

Racial or Ethnic Group	Genetic Disorder	Inheritance
Mediterranean (Italian, Greek, North African)	β-Thalassemia	AR
	Glucose-6-phosphatate dehydrogenase deficiency	XLR
Middle Eastern	β-Thalassemia	AR
	Familial Mediterranean fever	AR
Portuguese	Machado-Joseph disease	AR
Puerto Rican	Hermansky-Pudlak syndrome	AR
Southeast Asians	α-Thalassemia	AR
	β-Thalassemia	AR

AD, autosomal dominant; AR, autosomal recessive; XLR, X-linked recessive.

■ SUMMARY

A family history is essential in the diagnosis and management of birth defects, genetic disorders, and diseases for which there is a genetic predisposition.[4] The information obtained is useful for anticipatory guidance, appropriate health screening, and counseling regarding reproductive risks. However, as good a tool as family history is, it is only good if done well, and updated regularly.

REFERENCES

1. Bennett RL. *The Practical Guide to the Genetic Family History*. 2nd ed. Hoboken, NJ: Wiley-Blackwell; 2010.

2. Dolan SM, Moore C. Linking family history in obstetric and pediatric care: assessing risk for genetic disease and birth defects. *Pediatrics*. 2007;120(suppl 2):S66-S70.

3. Solomon BD, Jack B, Feero WG. The clinical content of preconception care: genetics and genomics. *Am J Obstet Gynecol*. 2008;199:S340-S344.

4. Committee on Genetics. Committee opinion—family history as a risk assessment tool. *Obstetrics & Gynecology*. 2011;117:747-750.

RESOURCES

The American Medical Association has a pamphlet available online entitled "Family Medical History in Disease Prevention (http://www.ama-assn.org/ama1/pub/upload/mm/464/family_history02.pdf).

The National Society of Genetic Counselors has available a guide for constructing a family history which is family friendly. (http://www.nsgc.org/Publications/ShopNSGC/tabid/55/pid/33/default.aspx).

The U.S. Department of Health and Human Services through the Surgeons General's Family Health History Initiative makes available "My Family Health Portrait Tool" which can be used by families to create a family history (https://familyhistory.hhs.gov).

CHAPTER 5

Principles of Genetic Counseling

Although there have been many attempts to define what it means to provide genetic counseling, the provision of genetic counseling is a process that needs to vary depending on the specific clinical circumstances. In the case of a patient seeking genetic counseling because of a cousin with cystic fibrosis, the components of the session likely will include a discussion of the natural history of cystic fibrosis, an explanation of autosomal recessive inheritance, the risk the patient and her partner are carriers of the gene, and finally a summary of available testing to determine their exact carrier status. Prior to providing them in depth information, a complete medical, family, and social history would be obtained to determine if there are other factors that could impact a future pregnancy.[1] Counseling in this circumstance should be nondirective; that is, the counselor provides the information necessary for the individual or couple to make informed decisions. This type of counseling is important, especially in a circumstance where both members of the couple are subsequently found to be carriers of the cystic fibrosis gene. The reproductive options available to them should be explained to them fully, and without bias. These options will range from not having children to preimplantation genetic diagnosis. The role of the counselor (whether that is a trained genetics professional or a general obstetrician-gynecologist) is to provide an explanation of each option, including the risks and benefits of each approach. There is no place for the provision of "recommendation."

On the other hand, providing genetic counseling to a 35-year-old woman that has just been found to carry a BRCA-1 mutation is likely to include precise information on current recommendations regarding prophylactic mastectomy and oophorectomy. The role of the counselor is to recognize when there are clear evidence-based guidelines, and when the options presented to the patient allow her to make a decision based on having balanced and complete information.

The following cases outline the importance of obtaining a complete family history, understanding patterns of inheritance, and using that information to calculate the risks involved, and knowing the various testing options available to the individual or couple.

Case 1: At the time of her annual visit your 26-year-old nulligravida patient tells you that she and her husband have decided they want to start their family. However, she is concerned because her first cousin died at age 3 of Tay-Sachs disease.

The key to providing appropriate counseling to patients regarding their risk for genetic disorders is obtaining a complete family history, and using that information to assess the potential risk to the patient or her offspring.[2] Although there are many ways to obtain family history information, the most effective approach for both obtaining the information and assessing the risk is a three-generation pedigree, as depicted in Figure 5-1. As noted in Chapter 4, a simple pedigree uses the following symbols: squares for males, circles for females, and by small filled in circles for miscarriages. Individuals with a genetic disease have their square or circle filled in, and a slash through the symbol indicates the person has died. Spouses are connected by a horizontal line and children connected to their parents by vertical lines. Ages can be added if that information is key to interpretation (eg, early-onset breast cancer). Ethnic backgrounds of both sides of the family should be documented.

In Figure 5-1 we have used the question mark to represent a potential future pregnancy. Your patient, known as the proband, is designated by the arrow. The first step in the analysis of risk is to ascertain the inheritance of the disease within the family. In this case scenario Tay-Sachs is an autosomal recessive disease, one that occurs because the affected individual has two copies of the mutated gene, one copy inherited from each of his parents. His parents, who carry one mutated gene and one normal gene, are described as "carriers." Because the patient's uncle

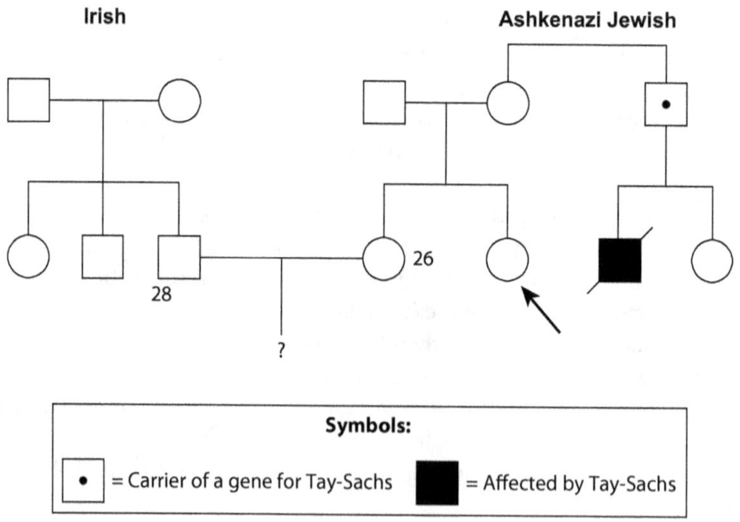

FIGURE 5-1. Pedigree for Case 1.

is a carrier of the Tay-Sachs mutation, one of his parents also must be a carrier. Therefore, your patient's mother could have received either the mutated gene or the normal gene from that parent, giving her a 50% chance of being a carrier. Likewise, if she did receive the Tay-Sachs gene, she has a 50% chance of passing it to her daughter, giving your patient a one in four chance (25%) that she carries the Tay-Sachs gene. Table 5-1 provides the risk figures for various relationships when dealing with autosomal recessive disorders.

However, your patient is only at risk for having a child with Tay-Sachs disease if her husband also carries the gene. There is no history of Tay-Sachs disease in his family so we must determine the likelihood that he is a carrier from population studies. It is known that certain ethnic groups (Ashkenazi Jews, French-Canadians) have a high carrier frequency (approximately one in 30 individuals from these ethnic groups carry the mutation). Individuals from other ethnic groups have a much lower carrier frequency (~1 in 300), and it is important to remember that anyone, regardless of ethnicity, can be a carrier for disorders, like Tay-Sachs, that are often identified with a specific ethnic group.

Now that we have determined the likelihood that each member of the couple is a carrier (one in four for your patient and 1 in 300 for her spouse), it is possible to tell them exactly their risk for having a child with Tay-Sachs disease. For autosomal recessive disorders, if both parents are carriers of the mutation, they have a 25% (one-fourth) chance of having a child that gets a mutated gene from each parent. Therefore, the risk that your patient will have an affected child is the risk she is a carrier (1/4) times the risk her husband is a carrier (1/300) times the risk of an affected child if they are both carriers (1/4), giving them a risk of one in 4800. Although their risk is relatively low, it is substantially higher than their risk without a positive family history (one in 36,000). At this point the next step in providing genetic counseling is a thorough discussion of the various testing options to better refine the true likelihood that one or both of the couple is a carrier of the Tay-Sachs gene. In practice a referral to a genetic professional to discuss the options of carrier testing would be appropriate. Further chapters of this book will provide an overview of the various approaches to testing.

■ TABLE 5-1. Risk of Being a Tay-Sachs (TS) Carrier with a Positive Family History		
If the Following Family Member	**Has TS**	**Is a TS Carrier**
Parent	1	1 in 2
Sibling	2 in 3	1 in 2
Aunt/Uncle	1 in 3	1 in 4
Niece/Nephew	1 in 2	1 in 4
First cousin	1 in 4	1 in 8

These figures only consider risk based on genetic contributions from the side of the family with a positive history. Additional risk may be inherited from the other side of the family.

Case 2: At the time of her first prenatal appointment at 8 weeks' gestation, a 30-year-old primagravida indicates that her maternal uncle died from complications of hemophilia.

Figure 5-2 depicts the patient's family history in a pedigree format. Although it will be essential to know what form of hemophilia (A or B) the uncle had for future diagnostic testing, both forms of hemophilia are inherited as X-linked recessive disorders. Because the gene is located on the X chromosome, a mutation on one X in a female has no clinical significance; she is said to be a carrier. On the other hand, the presence of that same mutation on the X chromosome of a male results in the disorder, as males have only one X-chromosome. X-linked recessive disorders are recognized by family histories showing only affected males, and no male to male transmission (fathers only pass a Y-chromosome to their sons).

In assessing the risk for this patient we must assume that her uncle does not represent a new mutation (relatively rare in hemophilia), and therefore his mother is a carrier of the hemophilia gene. Our patient's mother thus would have a 50% (1/2) chance of being a carrier for the hemophilia gene, resulting in a 25% chance our patient also carries the mutation. She can either pass the X-chromosome with the mutation, or the X-chromosome she received from her father (no mutation) to her sons. Our analysis of this family history indicates a one in eight chance that the patient's sons will have hemophilia. As noted above, further evaluation will require knowing if possible, the specific type of hemophilia the uncle had, and this information will direct the type of molecular testing necessary for determining if

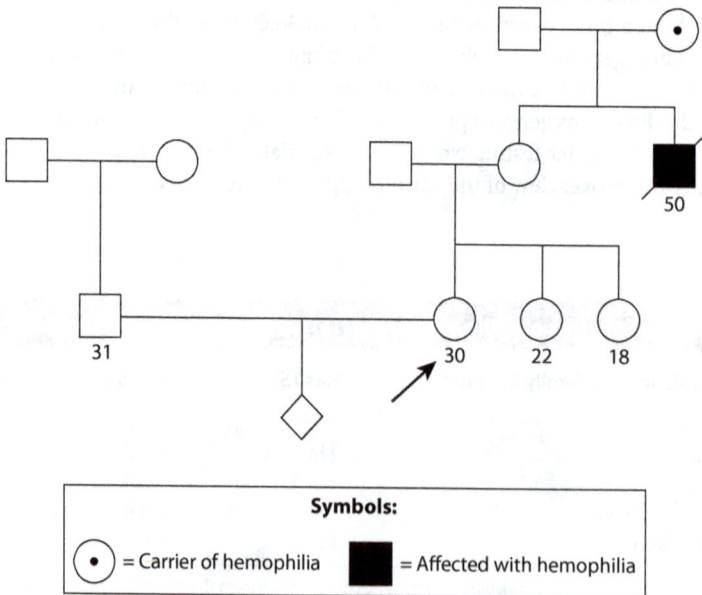

FIGURE 5-2. Pedigree for Case 2.

this patient carries the mutation for hemophilia. This case also represents both the opportunity and dilemma we face with an inherited disease in the family. The patient's two younger sisters are at similar risk for having children affected with hemophilia. She must be encouraged to share the counseling information with her family members in order for them to make informed reproductive decisions. The dilemma arises in families where estrangement or other dysfunction prevents communication between family members.

> **Case 3: A 30-year-old patient presents to you for preconception counseling. She had one previous pregnancy with a different partner that ended in miscarriage. Her medical history is completely negative, and she takes no medication. Her family history is remarkable for a brother, age 15 with a recent diagnosis of Marfan syndrome. Her father died last year of heart disease.**

Figure 5-3 depicts in a pedigree format the family history of this patient. Her previous relationship that resulted in a miscarriage is shown. The slash through the horizontal line indicates that she no longer is in a relationship with this person. Her father died at age 70 of "heart disease," and her mother is living without health issues at age 55. Her brother has a known inherited condition, Marfan syndrome, which is inherited in an autosomal dominant fashion. A single copy of the mutated gene results in the disorder, and both males and females are affected. However, individuals who inherit the mutated gene can vary significantly in the physical expression of the disease (phenotype). This variation in presentation, which can occur within family members inheriting the same genetic mutation, is termed variable expressivity. For certain autosomal dominant disorders, some individuals who inherit the mutated gene have no physical characteristics at all, and in this situation the gene is termed "nonpenetrant." Penetrance of a gene is calculated based on population information; how many people known to have the gene (such as someone with an affected parent and an affected child) have no physical manifestation of the mutation.

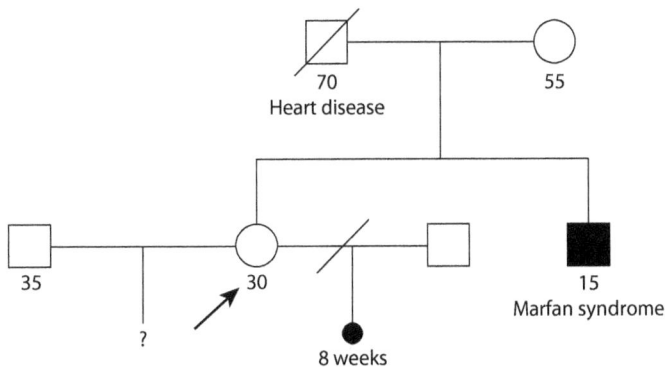

FIGURE 5-3. Pedigree for Case 3.

Autosomal dominant conditions have another characteristic that may complicate the counseling provided. New mutations are common in many dominant disorders, and new dominant mutations are associated with advanced paternal age. In this family history we have two possible clues. First, her father died of "heart disease." Was the heart disease a ruptured aortic aneurysm, a common cause of death in individuals with Marfan syndrome? Was his body habitus consistent with that expected for someone with Marfan syndrome? Secondly, based on when the patient's father died, he was approximately 56 years old when he fathered the patient's brother (advanced paternal age). Therefore, based on the pedigree we have a risk that the patient has Marfan syndrome varying from 50% (her father is affected) to 0% (her brother is a new mutation). Her physical examination may allow a better refinement of the risk, but an evaluation by a clinical geneticist, and appropriate molecular testing will be necessary to provide a more precise diagnosis, and further discussion regarding the risk of pregnancy for the patient, and her likelihood of having an affected child.

These scenarios illustrate the importance of genetic counseling in the most common circumstance in the practice of the obstetrician-gynecologist—the preconception visit and the first prenatal visit. A solid knowledge of the common patterns of inheritance is the basis for providing accurate and complete information to one's patients. In addition, a knowledge of those situations that should prompt a referral to a genetics professional is essential. An excellent resource is Pletcher et al.[3]

REFERENCES

1. Solomon BD, Jack B, Feero WG. The clinical content of preconception care: genetics and genomics. *Am J Obstet Gynecol.* 2008;199:S340-S344.
2. Bennett RL. The family medical history as a tool in preconception consultation. *J Community Genet.* 2012;3:175-183.
3. Pletcher BA, Toriello HV, Hoblin SJ, et al. Indications for genetic referral: a guide for health care professionals. *Gent Med.* 2007;9:385-389.

Clinical Genetics in Obstetrics and Gynecology

Preconception Counseling

Case 1: Ms. Meckel is a 25-year-old whose first and only pregnancy ended in a full-term normally grown infant with a large skin-covered encephalocele. The infant died a few hours after birth which, she was told, was the result of undeveloped lungs. Her family history, as well as her husband's, is negative for a history of neural tube defects, or any other birth defects. Likewise, there is no history of early infant death in any family members. Ms. Meckel believes an autopsy was performed,

but she has never seen a report, or been told the results of the autopsy. She would like to have a child, but is concerned about the risk she will have another child with the same condition. How would you counsel this patient?

For a couple at risk for having a child with a genetic disorder there are a number of reproductive options: (1) choosing to remain childless, (2) having children and accepting the risk, (3) choosing to have prenatal diagnosis to determine if the fetus is affected, (4) having artificial insemination or oocyte donation to avoid passing on the mutant gene, (5) undergoing preimplantation genetic diagnosis (PGD), or (6) adoption. In order to have all these options available to them, a couple must receive counseling regarding their specific risks before becoming pregnant; thus, the term preconception counseling.

A preconception counseling session should include a detailed family history and construction of a pedigree. Medical records should be obtained, if necessary, to confirm a diagnosis. Complete medical histories of both members of the couple should be ascertained. Should a significant factor be found, the information provided should include the risk of occurrence in their offspring, the natural history of the disorder, and the testing available to them. Counseling should always be done in a nondirective fashion.

Preconception counseling is the responsibility of all obstetrician-gynecologists, but it is also their responsibility to remain current on diagnostic tests available to determine carrier status or for prenatal diagnosis. Because genetics is a rapidly changing field, each practitioner should have a good working relationship with the local genetics center, and refer couples for consultation, when the situation requires more in-depth knowledge of the disorder, there is an undiagnosed disorder, or when more specialized testing is necessary.

The purpose of this chapter will be to discuss those circumstances in which preconception genetic counseling is appropriate. Table 6-1 briefly outlines the family history, medical history, and social history factors that may require a preconception counseling session. Although it is possible to elicit these findings by careful history taking, a more cost-effective approach is to use a questionnaire such as the one offered by the American College of Obstetricians and Gynecologists (ACOG). In addition to a questionnaire, it is important to ask a general question such as: "Is there any child that died unexpectedly, any person who has a learning disability or is 'slow,' or is there any disease that seems to run in the family?" It is common for a couple to check "no" for family members with mental retardation, even when further evaluation reveals several members with moderate to severe intellectual disability. In these families, such individuals are not labeled as mentally retarded, but as "slow" or "learning disabled." This type of question also will illicit the history of the family member who died in early childhood as a result of a metabolic disease.

▪ TABLE 6-1. Common Indications for Preconception Genetic Consultation

Previous pregnancy history
   Fetal demise
   Recurrent pregnancy loss
Previous child with a genetic disorder
   Chromosomal: Down syndrome
   Structural: dwarfism, neural tube defect
   Metabolic: neonatal or early childhood death, ambiguous genitalia
   Hematologic: anemia, bleeding disorder
   Mental retardation
Family history of a genetic disorder
   Bleeding disorders: hemophilia
   Neurologic disease: muscular dystrophy, myotonic dystrophy
   Mental retardation: fragile (X) syndrome
   Cystic fibrosis
Ethnic origin from population at high risk of genetic disorder
   Ashkenazi Jewish: Tay-Sachs disease
   French-Canadian: Tay-Sachs disease
   African-American: sickle cell anemia
   Mediterranean: β-thalassemia
   Asian: α-thalassemia and β-thalassemia
Maternal medical disorders
   Diabetes
   Phenylketonuria
Maternal medications
   Anticonvulsants
   Lithium
   Accutane
   Any chronically used medication
Socially used drugs
   Alcohol
   Cocaine

▪ PREVIOUS PREGNANCY HISTORY

A history of a previous stillbirth should prompt a review of the pregnancy records, as well as the autopsy report, if one was performed. The patient's recollection most often does not provide adequate or complete information on which to base counseling. For example, a stillborn with an encephalocele could represent an isolated neural tube defect (NTD) with a 2% to 3% risk of recurrence, or a component of a number of genetic syndromes, some of which have a 25% risk of recurrence. The patient with an isolated NTD will benefit from preconceptional folate supplementation, but the risk of recurrence will not be modified by folate, if the disorder is a genetic syndrome with autosomal recessive inheritance.

Recurrent miscarriages always should raise suspicion of a possible genetic or chromosomal etiology (see Chapter 14). However, two points must be emphasized. First, a translocation or other chromosome rearrangement will be found as the etiology of recurrent miscarriage in approximately 3% to 6% of cases.[1] Second, the history of a normal child interposed in a history of multiple losses should not be taken as a reason to rule out a chromosomal etiology. An individual who carries a balanced translocation would be expected to have three possible gametes: (1) those with the unbalanced form of the translocation, (2) those with the balanced form of the translocation, and (3) those that did not receive the translocation at all. The latter two types of gametes would be expected to result in normal offspring.

The first priority is to obtain the autopsy report. In this circumstance, the combination of findings were a skin-covered encephalocele, polydactyly, and large polycystic kidneys. The autopsy is consistent with Meckel-Gruber syndrome, an autosomal recessive disorder. You would counsel the patient that the risk of recurrence is 25% for any subsequent pregnancy. When a specific diagnosis is made of a mendelian disorder, the next step should be consultation with a geneticist to determine if a specific gene mutation has been found for the disorder. If there is a known mutation, then the patient has the option of PGD, or prenatal diagnosis by chorionic villus sampling (CVS). If a specific mutation has not been identified, a second trimester ultrasound may be diagnostic, if known structural malformations are present. Although the features of Meckel-Gruber may be variable, at least one of the triad of abnormalities should be present in a subsequent affected pregnancy. Should ultrasound be the only option available, prenatal evaluation in a subsequent pregnancy always should be done by sonologists with extensive experience in detecting fetal structural malformations.

Finally, although folate supplementation (1 mg) is recommended for all women planning a pregnancy, this patient would not be a candidate for the 4 mg dose recommended for women who have had a pregnancy complicated by an NTD. Folate supplementation will not decrease the risk of an NTD that is part of a mendelian syndrome.

> **Case 2: Mr. and Mrs. Rimoin present to you for a preconception counseling session. They have one child together, a son, who has been diagnosed with achondroplasia. Mr. Rimoin has a second child with a previous partner who also has achondroplasia. Mr. and Mrs. Rimoin are 6 ft 4 in and 5 ft 11 in, respectively. There are no other family members on either side of the family that have short stature, or dwarfism. Mr. Rimoin is very concerned about the possibility of another child with achondroplasia, and wants an explanation as to why he has had two children with an autosomal dominant condition when his height is normal. How would you approach the counseling for this couple?**

■ PREVIOUS CHILD WITH A GENETIC DISORDER

The most common way to ascertain a couple at risk for a genetic disorder is by the previous birth of an affected child. For some disorders, the history will be obtained when taking a pregnancy history that reveals a child born with a birth defect. But for later onset diseases, further information may be ascertained only if the history taking includes questions such as: "What is the child's health now?," "Has the child had any significant health problems?," "Is the child on any special diets or medications?" Many of the degenerative neurologic diseases may not present clinically until age 2 years or later, and may not be seen as a birth defect by the family. A child placed on appropriate dietary management at birth for a metabolic disorder, such as phenylketonuria (PKU), and doing well at age 4 may not be considered by the couple to have a genetic disease. For most of these disorders, the inheritance pattern is autosomal recessive, with a 25% recurrence risk. More importantly, prenatal diagnosis is possible in the majority of these conditions. Even in cases in which an effective treatment exists, many couples will choose prenatal testing for reassurance, if the fetus is unaffected, and for planning if the fetus is affected. It is the obstetrician's responsibility to inform the couple of all of the options available to them.

One of the major difficulties facing the practicing obstetrician/gynecologists is the rapidity with which discoveries are occurring in the field of genetics, and the major impact new information can have for counseling patients at risk. One of the best examples is that of a couple with a previous child having achondroplasia. This common form of dwarfism is inherited in an autosomal dominant fashion; therefore, an individual with achondroplasia has a 50% chance of having a child with the same disorder. Because the gene is 100% penetrant, an individual has the disease if the gene is present. Parents of normal height, who have a child with achondroplasia, should be expected to have essentially a zero chance of a second child because the first child must represent a new mutation in a sperm or egg. In addition, our counseling to the couple would have, in the past, included information that the disorder could not be detected prenatally by ultrasound until the third trimester. As more couples who had been counseled regarding this low risk had a second child with achondroplasia, it became clear that another mechanism must be found to explain what appeared to be a 5% risk of recurrence in these couples. With the advent of molecular studies, mutational analysis confirmed that a second affected child within a family had the exact mutation seen in the previously affected sibling. The mechanism to explain this finding is germ cell mosaicism (Figure 6-1). Depending on where in the lineage of the egg or sperm the mutation occurred, the number of gametes with the mutation could range from a single gamete to 100% of the gametes. Because of multiple DNA replications that occur in the formation of sperm, almost all cases of new dominant mutations are paternal in origin.

The discovery that the mutation causing achondroplasia is in the gene for fibroblast growth factor 3 allows the very precise diagnosis of achondroplasia as early

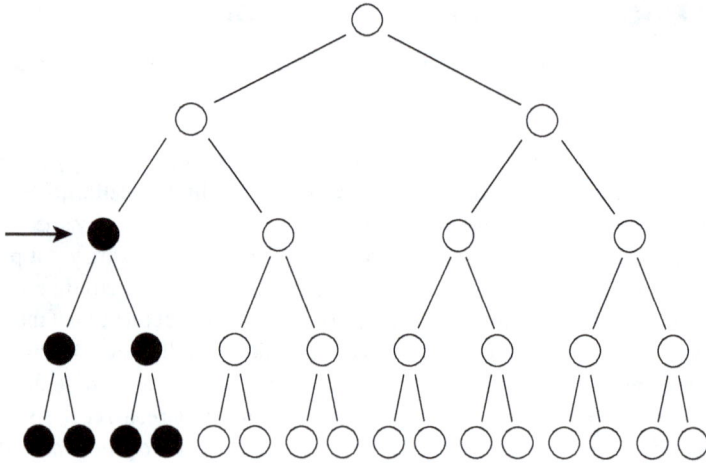

FIGURE 6-1. Schematic representation of a mutation in the formation of sperm (arrow) resulting in germline mosaicism for a new mutation.

as the first trimester with CVS or by cell free fetal DNA in the maternal circulation (see Chapters 8 and 9).[2] Preimplantation diagnosis is an option as well.

■ FAMILY HISTORY OF A GENETIC DISORDER

Analysis of a family history to determine if a couple is at risk for a child with a genetic disorder requires not only a basic knowledge of principles of mendelian inheritance, but also a current knowledge of what genetic conditions are diagnosable prenatally. This area is one in which a good collaborative relationship with a local genetics community is essential.

The classic example of the importance of family history is that of an X-linked disorder such as hemophilia or muscular dystrophy, on the maternal side of the family. In traditional X-linked inheritance only males are affected. Females, who have two X chromosomes, are carriers of the disorder. In a pedigree, such as Figure 6-2, the proband (designated by the arrow) is concerned about her risk of having a child with hemophilia B (factor IX deficiency). Pedigree analysis allows a calculation of her risk of being a carrier, which would be 1/4. If she were a carrier, her chance of an affected child would be 1/4 (1/2 chance of passing an affected chromosome X and a 1/2 chance it will be a male). Therefore, by multiplying her risk of being a carrier times 1/4, we can calculate the chance this patient would have a son with hemophilia (1/16). Until a few years ago the only options for a couple who chose to be pregnant would be: (1) accept the risk, or (2) choose prenatal diagnosis to determine the sex of the fetus and carry only female fetuses. With modern molecular techniques, it is possible to determine an individual's carrier status. By completing these family studies before conception, a couple can make informed decisions regarding testing, if the proband carries the gene, or can

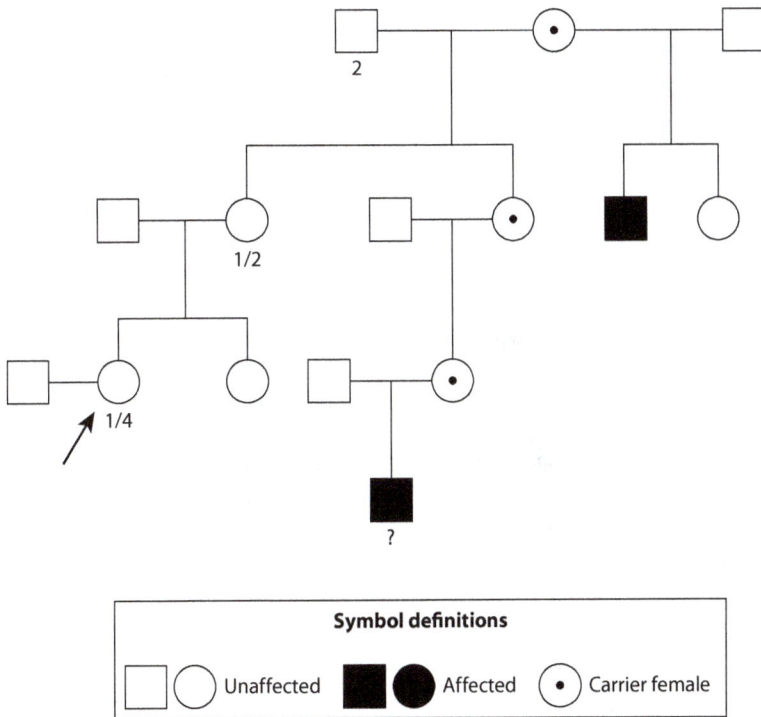

FIGURE 6-2. Pedigree of family with several males affected with hemophilia B, depicted by shaded squares. Proband is designated by arrow.

undertake pregnancy with the knowledge that the child would not be at risk, if she is not a carrier.

A family history of a recessive disorder generally does not place a couple at a significant risk of having an affected child, unless the carrier frequency of that disorder is quite common in the population. For instance, if a history is taken in which the husband has a nephew with phenylketonuria, we can calculate that his risk of being a carrier is 1/2. To determine his wife's chance of being a carrier, we must know the frequency of the disease in the population, and in the case of PKU, this figure is 1 per 10,000 live births. Therefore, the wife's chance of being a carrier would be 1/50 (two times the square root of the disease incidence). If both individuals were carriers, their chance for an affected child would be 1/4. Hence, for this couple the risk of having a child with PKU would be 1/400 (1/2 × 1/50 × 1/4).

However, a disease that is much more prevalent in the general population will have a much higher carrier frequency. In the case of cystic fibrosis where the carrier frequency is 1 in 29, the risk for a couple, such as the couple above, would be 1/232 (1/2 × 1/29 × 1/4). In the case of recessive disorders carrier testing, if available, should be offered to better define the risk the couple has for having a child with the disease in question.

A history of mental retardation in the family offers one of the more complex counseling sessions because of the myriad of causes for mental retardation. Unless the affected individual is an isolated case of mental retardation and a distant relative of the pregnancy at risk, it is essential to obtain medical records to determine, if possible, the specific etiology. Once an etiology is established, the inheritance pattern will generally be known, and a risk figure can be established for the couple. The one disease to always keep foremost in the differential diagnosis is the fragile-X syndrome (see Chapters 3 and 14 for a discussion of fragile-X).

In counseling families with a previously affected child or a family history of a specific genetic disorder, a precise diagnosis is essential. Once the diagnosis is known, inheritance patterns can be discussed with family, and options for testing by PGD or prenatal diagnosis can be outlined. For Mr. and Mrs. Rimoin the information outlined in the above discussion on achondroplasia should be presented in lay terms, and a plan for pregnancy management should be developed. Referral will depend on whether the family desires more detailed information about the various testing options.

■ ETHNIC ORIGIN FROM POPULATION AT HIGH RISK FOR A GENETIC DISORDER

When assessing the medical and family history of a couple planning to undertake a pregnancy, it is important to elicit information regarding the ethnic origin of each member of the couple. Several ethnic groups have a relatively high carrier frequency for certain genetic disorders. For example, an individual of Ashkenazic Jewish heritage (almost 90% of individuals who identify themselves of Jewish ethnicity) has a 1/30 chance of being a carrier for Tay-Sachs disease, a severe degenerative neurologic disease, causing death in early childhood. Because Tay-Sachs disease is an autosomal recessive disease, both parents must be carriers in order to have an affected child. Preconception screening for couples of Jewish heritage is the recommended approach.

Two other circumstances that often arise are (1) one member of the couple has only one parent who is Jewish, and (2) one member of the couple is Jewish, and the other is not. In the first instance the individual with only one Jewish parent still has a 1/60 chance of being a carrier of Tay-Sachs, and should be offered screening. In the second circumstance, it must be remembered that the Tay-Sachs gene also occurs in non-Jewish individuals, but at a much lower incidence (1/300). Therefore, the pregnancy of a couple where only one member is of Jewish heritage remains at a significant risk for a child with Tay-Sachs disease. At the very least, the person of Jewish ancestry should be screened, and if that person is a carrier, the non-Jewish person should be screened.

Other ethnic groups at risk for genetic disorders for which there are good screening tests available are: Asians (α-thalassemia, β-thalassemia), Mediterraneans (β-thalassemia), African-Americans (sickle cell disease), and French-Canadians

(Tay-Sachs disease). A simple first line screen for the thalassemias is a complete blood count with indices. Individuals who carry either the alpha or beta thalassemia gene have a mild anemia and a low mean corpuscular volume (MCV). An MCV of less than 80 femtoliters should prompt an evaluation of possible carrier status for these hematologic diseases (see Chapter 3 for a more complete discussion of thalassemia).

> **Case 3: Ms. Brambati is a 28-year-old attorney who presents to your office for a preconception counseling visit. She has no previous pregnancies, has had regular 28-day cycles since onset of menses at age 12. Her only medical problem is an idiopathic seizure disorder that had its onset in early childhood. Her seizures are well controlled by valproic acid therapy. She takes no other medication except a daily prenatal vitamin. She does not smoke or drink. Her family history, and that of her spouse are both negative for any birth defects, genetic conditions, or other factors that should increase the risk to a pregnancy. Both she and her husband are of Italian ancestry.**

■ MATERNAL MEDICAL DISORDERS

Certain medical conditions in the mother may increase the risk for congenital malformations in that individual's offspring. The most well-recognized disease in this category is maternal insulin-dependent diabetes. Patients with poor glucose control during the time of organogenesis have a two- to threefold higher risk of birth defects in their offspring than patients without diabetes. Good glucose control initiated before conception appears to diminish the risk of birth defects to a level comparable to that of the normal population.

A less well-recognized situation is the risk of maternal PKU. One of the major triumphs of genetic screening is the newborn screening program for PKU. A child affected with PKU is unable to metabolize phenylalanine, and the resulting high serum levels result in central nervous system damage and severe mental retardation. However, institution of a low phenylalanine diet within a few days of birth normalizes serum phenylalanine levels, and the child will develop normally with normal intelligence. Until recently, dietary restriction was discontinued when the child reached adolescence, because it was thought that high serum phenylalanine levels were not harmful to the "mature" brain.

The success of PKU screening has resulted in a number of women with PKU having now reached child-bearing age. Because PKU is a recessively inherited condition the risk for having a child with PKU is quite low. However, in the woman who is no longer on a phenylalanine restricted diet, the serum levels of phenylalanine are quite high, and phenylalanine easily crosses the placenta. Thus, the developing brain, heart, and other organs are exposed to very high levels of phenylalanine potentially resulting in a child with severe mental retardation, microcephaly, congenital heart defects, and intrauterine growth restriction.

Even though the child does not have PKU, the disease that results from the mother's high serum levels of phenylalanine is as devastating as PKU itself.

Although the number of patients with good dietary control is still small, the published data are highly suggestive that normalizing serum phenylalanine levels before conception results in children with normal intelligence and without a higher risk for other birth defects.[3]

■ MATERNAL MEDICATIONS

One of the most easily preventable causes of congenital malformations is the group of birth defects caused by exposure to teratogens. However, these malformations are only preventable if the medication or environmental exposure is discontinued before the patient conceives. The problem of medication exposure to the fetus is substantial. The average number of medications used in the first trimester is 2.6 with over 80% of women using at least one medication. More than 25% of pregnant women used 4 or more medications in the first trimester.[4] Preconception counseling can have its most significant benefit in this area. It is beyond the scope of this chapter to cover the topic of teratology in depth, but some commonly used medications will be discussed.

Anticonvulsants

Hydantoins are the most widely studied of the anticonvulsant drugs. It is generally accepted that there is a fetal hydantoin syndrome seen in a significant number of children born to mothers taking hydantoins in the first trimester. The features seen include subtle dysmorphic facial features, cleft lip/palate, congenital heart defects, and developmental delay. Some features of the fetal hydantoin syndrome may be seen in as many as 30% of children exposed in the first trimester.[5] The risk of major malformations is 2 to 3 times higher than in unexposed pregnancies.[6]

Valproic acid is another commonly used medication for the treatment of seizures. Although there have been reports of a fetal valproate syndrome with features quite similar to those of hydantoin, one of the major teratogenic risk of valproic acid appears to involve the development of the lower spine. Approximately 1% of infants exposed in the first trimester will have a lower lumbo-sacral myelomeningocele.[7] Overall, valproic acid appears to have the highest risk of causing fetal malformation among the antiepileptic medications. In addition, fetal exposure to valproic acid has been shown to significantly increase the risk of autism spectrum disorders.[8] However, the absolute risk for autism is less than 5%, and, like the risk for spina bifida, it should be a part of the counseling about the risks and benefits of continuing, or stopping, the valproic acid before attempting pregnancy.

For the patient planning a pregnancy the optimal approach is to discontinue medications before conception, especially if she has been seizure free for 2 or more years, has a normal neurologic exam, and a normal electroencephalogram, and is without complicating factors such as known central nervous abnormalities. If the patient remains seizure-free without medications, the pregnancy can be undertaken without concerns. The most important component to the management of the patient with a seizure disorder is a coordinated approach, between the patient's neurologist and her obstetrician/gynecologist, that effectively manages her seizures with the least risk to her anticipated pregnancy.

Isotretinoin (Accutane)

One of the most potent teratogens on the market today is Accutane, a medication widely used for the treatment of a variety of dermatologic conditions. It has devastating effects on the developing brain and heart, and is associated with the very unique malformation of absence of the external ear. The risk of malformations after exposure in the first trimester is approximately 25%. Preconception counseling for the patient being treated with Accutane should include a recommendation that the medication be stopped well in advance of becoming pregnant, because of the long half-life of this particular medication.

Lithium

For the treatment of bipolar disorders, lithium is a very effective agent. Therefore, the obstetrician/gynecologist is likely to have a number of patients on this medication. Older registry-based studies suggested quite a significant risk (10%) for fetal cardiac defects after exposures to lithium in the first trimester. A prospective study suggested a much lower risk (1%), but the abnormality seen (the Ebstein anomaly) is quite rare in nonexposed patients, suggesting that lithium is indeed a teratogen.[9] However, current studies suggest a much lower risk of the Ebstein anomaly (0.01%-0.05%, compared to the population risk of 0.005%).[10] Given that the alternative treatments for bipolar affective disorders are the antiepileptic drugs, such as valproic acid, that have a risk of malformation ranging from 2.7% to 8.7%, lithium remains the best option for treatment during pregnancy.

■ SOCIALLY USED DRUGS

Malformations that result from socially used substances theoretically should be entirely preventable through preconception counseling. Unfortunately, a large proportion of women who would benefit from this form of counseling will not seek medical care until pregnancy has already occurred, and often is well advanced.

Alcohol

Of all the socially used drugs, alcohol is the most significant in terms of numbers of pregnancies exposed. More than half of women use alcohol at some point in their pregnancy. Therefore, it should not be a surprising statistic that fetal alcohol exposure is one of the leading causes of intellectual disability. Significant alcohol use over the course of pregnancy results in a full spectrum of malformations, including prenatal and/or postnatal growth restriction, microcephaly, facial dysmorphic features, and mental deficiency/developmental delay. There is at present no consensus on a threshold amount of alcohol that is associated with fetal effects. The safest choice is to avoid alcohol consumption following conception.

On the other hand, there is no information to suggest a significant risk associated with an occasional drink during pregnancy; information that will be reassuring to the patient who had a "social" drink early in an unsuspected pregnancy.

■ NUTRITIONAL SUPPLEMENTS

Approximately 40% of women of childbearing age supplement their diets with vitamins or mineral preparations.[11] The finding that folate supplementation reduces the risk of neural tube defects has resulted in an increased consumption of this supplement, and therefore, a note of caution must be raised. Two representative examples are outlined to emphasize both the positive and the negative aspects of vitamin and mineral supplementation.

Folic Acid

The effectiveness of folic acid supplementation in preventing recurrence of neural tube defects opened a new area where preconceptional counseling has a dramatic impact. Neural tube defects (spina bifida, anencephaly, encephalocele) are among the most common birth defects, occurring in 1 to 2 of every 1000 live births. The risk of recurrence in a subsequent pregnancy after the birth of a child with an NTD is 2% to 3%, suggesting multifactorial inheritance. This pattern of inheritance implies a combination of both genetic and environmental factors. One of the most significant environmental factors appears to be folate. In a prospective study of women receiving 4 mg of folate per day before conception, the risk of recurrence was reduced by almost 75%.[12] Other studies have shown a significant decrease in the occurrence (first case in a family) of neural tube defects in women using folate supplementation (0.4-0.8 mg) before and during the first 6 weeks of pregnancy.[13]

The present recommendations are that all women at increased risk (previous child with NTD or either parent with NTD) take 4 mg of folate per day beginning 1 month before conception, and continuing through the first 3 months of pregnancy. For women without risk factors the recommendation is 0.4 mg/d, not to exceed a total folate consumption of 1.0 mg/d. In the United States, folate now is added to breads and cereals. However, patients should be counseled that this fortification is not adequate to meet the recommendation, and they should be encouraged to take additional folate supplementation. In counseling women regarding the benefits of supplementation, it must be emphasized that there is no information to suggest that increasing the dosage will increase the benefit. On the contrary, increasing dosage could have detrimental effects, especially if the supplementation is in the form of a multivitamin preparation. For the woman who has a previous child with a NTD, it is essential that she be given a prescription for folate alone, and not attempt to achieve this dose by taking several prenatal vitamins. This approach would result in levels of other vitamins that would far exceed daily recommendations.

Despite the compelling data on the benefits of folic acid supplementation, a recent study found that only 31% of women were taking folic acid supplements prior to becoming pregnant. Among women less than age 20, the number taking supplements was 6%.[14] These dismal numbers suggest that additional food fortification with folic acid may be necessary to reach the level of prevention of NTD that is theoretically possible.

Vitamin A

Because of the medical benefits of vitamin A analogues in the treatment of dermatologic disorders, there has arisen a commercial industry touting the benefits of vitamin A supplementation for "blemish-free" skin. It now is quite common for women of childbearing age to be taking vitamin A supplementations at dosages well above the daily recommended allowance even for pregnancy. Adding to this, the amount in standard prenatal vitamins often will push the dosage well into the range that has been associated with a teratogenic effect (25,000 IU). One factor that complicates any recommendations being made is that current vitamin A supplements use β-carotene as the source of vitamin A. It appears to be a less potent form of vitamin A, and has not, to date, been associated with any teratogenic effect. However, if the patient is planning a pregnancy, the best advice is to not exceed recommended daily allowances of any vitamin or mineral.

Our case reflects a common dilemma faced by the obstetrician and the patient when the patient is being treated effectively for a medical condition, but with a medication known to cause fetal malformations. In the case of an anticonvulsant, the implication of stopping the medications is quite significant. Should the patient have a recurrence of her seizures, she may lose her license to drive as one very practical consequence of her decision to stop the medication. Switching medications may not be possible since many of the anticonvulsants are associated with an increase in fetal malformations. In some cases, the best course of action may be to continue the medication, and offer prenatal testing, such as ultrasound evaluation, to assess the fetal status. Any decision should be the result of an informed discussion with the patient, her neurologist, and other consultants that can provide appropriate input into the decision-making.

■ SUMMARY

The purpose of this chapter has not been to be all-inclusive, but to raise awareness of the benefits of preconception consultation in the prevention of birth defects. If there is to be a significant decrease in the incidence of congenital malformations, it will come only by intervention that occurs prior to organogenesis, and that opportunity is lost by the first prenatal visit.

REFERENCES

1. Franssen MTM, Korevaar JC, van der Veen F, et al. Reproductive outcome after chromosome analysis in couples with two or more miscarriages: case-control study. *BMJ.* 2006;332:759-763.
2. Shaing R, Thompson L, Zhu Y, et al. Mutations in the transmembrane domain of FGFR3 causes the most common genetic form of dwarfism, achondroplasia. *Cell.* 1994;78:335-342.

3. Prick BW, Hop WCJ, Duvekot JJ. Maternal phenylketonuria and hyperphenylalanin-emia in pregnancy: pregnancy complications and neonatal sequelae in untreated and treated pregnancies. *Am J Clin Nutr.* 2012;95:374-382.

4. Mitchell AA, Gilboa SM, Werler MM, et al. Medication use during pregnancy, with particular focus on prescription drugs: 1976-2008. *Am J Obstet Gynecol.* 2011;205:51. e1-51.e8.

5. Hanson JW, Myrianthopoulos NC, Harvey MAS, et al. Risks to the offspring of women treated with hydantoin anticonvulsants with emphasis on the fetal hydantoin syndrome. *J Pediatr.* 1976;89:662-668.

6. Meador KJ, Baker GA, Finnell RH, et al. In utero antiepileptic drug exposure: fetal death and malformations. *Neurology.* 2006;67:407-412.

7. Rosa FW. Spina bifida in infants of women treated with carbamazepine during pregnancy. *N Engl J Med.* 1991;324:674-677.

8. Christensen J, Gronbong TK, Sorensen MJ, et al. Prenatal valproate exposure and risk of autism spectrum disorders and childhood autism. *JAMA.* 2013;309: 1696-1703.

9. Jacobson SJ, Jones K, Johnson K, et al. Prospective multicenter study of pregnancy outcome after lithium exposure during the first trimester. *Lancet.* 1992;339:530-533.

10. Galbally M, Roberts M, Buist A. Mood stabilization in pregnancy: a systematic review. *Aust NZJ Psychiatry.* 2010;44:967-977.

11. Stewart ML, McDonald JT, Levy AS, et al. Vitamin/mineral supplement use: a tele-phone survey of adults in the United States. *J Am Diet Assoc.* 1985;85:1585-1590.

12. Milunsky A, Jick H, Jick S, et al. Multivitamin/folic acid supplementation in early pregnancy reduces the prevalence of neural tube defects. *JAMA.* 1989;262: 2847-2852.

13. Czeizel AE, Dudas I. Prevention of the first occurrence of neural tube defects by peri-conceptional vitamin supplementation. *N Engl J Med.* 1992;327:1832-1835.

14. Bestwick JP, Huttly WJ, Morris JK, Wald NJ. Prevention of neural tube defects: a cross-sectional study of the uptake of folic acid supplementation in nearly half a million women. *PLOS One.* 2014;9:1-6.

Common Chromosomal Abnormalities

- DOWN SYNDROME
- OTHER CHROMOSOMAL ABNORMALITIES
- CONCLUSION

Case 1: A 25-year-old patient presents to you for counseling. She underwent chorionic villus sampling and the chromosomal analysis revealed trisomy 21. How do you counsel your patient regarding the implication of this result?

DOWN SYNDROME

Trisomy 21 describes three copies of chromosome 21, but is often used interchangeably with Down syndrome (DS), the constellation of clinical findings that are the result of having one additional copy of chromosome 21. Its clinical features were first characterized by Landon Down in 1866, but the etiology of the syndrome was not recognized until 1959 by Lejeune and colleagues.[1] Trisomy 21 is the most common trisomy, occurring in approximately 1 in every 700 live births.[2] More than 95% cases of DS are the result of nondisjunction during meiosis, and most commonly meiosis I. Because of the strong association between maternal age and nondisjunction, the extra chromosome is maternal in origin in approximately 95% of cases. Of the remaining 5% of DS children, most will be the result of an unbalanced chromosome translocation. These translocations likewise result in three full copies of chromosome 21, and, thus, the term trisomy 21 can be used for both these forms of DS. In our case example, it would be essential to have the cytogenetic report before attempting to counsel the patient. Although the type of trisomy 21 has no

■ TABLE 7-1. Features of Trisomy 21

- Upslanted palpebral fissures
- Loose neck skin (extra skin fold)
- Flat nasal bridge
- Short anterior to posterior diameter of the head
- Epicanthal folds
- Single palmar crease
- Hypotonia

■ TABLE 7-2. Maternal Age and Down Syndrome Risk (Live Births)[3,4]

Maternal Age at Birth (Years)	Risk of Down Syndrome
20	1:1667
21	1:1667
22	1:1429
23	1:1429
24	1:1250
25	1:1250
26	1:1176
27	1:1111
28	1:1053
29	1:1000
30	1:952
31	1:909
32	1:769
33	1:602
34	1:482
35	1:375
36	1:289
37	1:224
38	1:173
39	1:136
40	1:106
41	1:82
42	1:63
43	1:49
44	1:38
45	1:30
46	1:23
47	1:18
48	1:14
49	1:11

implications for the clinical outcome of the child, the implication for future pregnancies, which will be discussed later, is significantly different.

When counseling a patient regarding DS, it is important to emphasize that infants with DS have few features that are recognizable to the lay person, and that the absence of significant morphologic features has no prognostic significance. Table 7-1 lists the features that are commonly seen in infants with DS. Of more importance for prognosis are the structural malformations that are associated with DS. Approximately 50% of children with DS will have a congenital heart defect, and of these cardiac defects the most common is an atrioventricular septal defect (endocardial cushion defect). However, ventricular septal defects, atrial septal defects, and tetralogy of Fallot are seen commonly in children with DS. Should the patient in our case study decide to continue her pregnancy, a fetal echocardiogram should be performed between 18 and 20 weeks' gestation to assess for fetal cardiac malformations.

Structural malformation of the gastrointestinal tract occurs in approximately 5% of DS children, the most common abnormality being duodenal atresia. The association between duodenal atresia and DS is significant. Of those cases of duodenal atresia detected in the fetus, 30% will be found to have DS. Other gastrointestinal malformations that are associated with DS include imperforate anus, tracheoesophageal fistula, other intestinal atresias, and Hirschsprung disease.

For most couples the most significant concern upon hearing the diagnosis of DS is the degree of intellectual disability. The majority of DS children will have moderate intellectual disability (IQ range of 30-60), but, as in all children, there is a range of IQ which can vary from mild to severe in its degree. Couples who are undecided about whether to continue a pregnancy with DS should be referred to a Down syndrome center or to a pediatrician with expertise in managing DS children in order to understand fully the overall prognosis for an individual with DS.

When counseling a couple who have had a child with DS, it is essential that the exact type of DS be known. In the case of trisomy 21, because of a nondisjunctional event, the empiric risk of recurrence in older studies was approximately 1%.[5] However, information from a large cytogenetic data set can be used to give more exact risks, depending on current age, and age at the time of the DS pregnancy.[6] In general terms, the risk for a patient under 30 to have a second affected child is 8.2X the age-specific risk for DS (see Table 7-2 for age specific risks for DS). For a patient over the age of 35, the risk is 1.7X the age-specific DS risk. If the DS is because of a balanced translocation, the parents must have chromosome studies to determine who carries the balanced form of the translocation. If the mother is the carrier, the risk of recurrence is 10%, whereas if the male has the translocation, the recurrence risk is 3% or less.

■ OTHER CHROMOSOMAL ABNORMALITIES

Trisomy 18 also is called Edwards syndrome, and occurs in approximately 1 in every 3000 live births. Like trisomy 21 it is associated with maternal age, but is more commonly due to nondisjunction in meiosis II.[7] Unlike trisomy 21, an extra chromosome 18 results in much more significant clinical implications. It is

> ■ **TABLE 7-3.** Features of Trisomy 18
>
> - Micrognathia (small jaw)
> - Low set malformed ears
> - Rocker bottom feet
> - Clenched hands
> - Hypoplastic thumbs

estimated that up to 98% of trisomy 18 conceptions end in spontaneous abortion. Of live born children, about one-half will die during the first week of life, and another 40% will die during the first year of life. However, approximately 10% will survive beyond 1 year of life, and may survive into late teens. Regardless of the length of survival the degree of intellectual disability is severe in all cases.

The constellation of malformations seen in trisomy 18 can be quite varied, but congenital heart defects, often complex in nature, are seen in up to 90% of infants. Table 7-3 outlines the common physical manifestations at birth in trisomy 18. In addition to the external features noted, gastrointestinal tract malformations and renal abnormalities are common in trisomy 18. Unlike trisomy 21, which rarely is associated with fetal growth restriction, trisomy 18 almost always has significant intrauterine growth restriction, often present in mid-trimester.

Trisomy 13 (Patau syndrome) occurs in one in every 5000 live births.[2] Similar to trisomy 18, up to 90% of infants with trisomy 13 will die in the first year of life, but survival into adulthood is not uncommon. It is associated with increasing maternal age, and most cases are the result of meiotic disjunction. However, because the 13;14 robertsonian translocation is common in the population (1 in 1000 individuals), trisomy 13 secondary to an unbalanced translocation accounts for up to 20% of children with the disorder.

The clinical manifestations of trisomy 13 are quite severe, with profound intellectual disability found in all survivors. The face and the brain are the common sites for malformations. Holoprosencephaly, cleft lip and palate, and microphthalmia (small eyes) are common abnormalities seen in infants with trisomy 13. Cardiac malformations are present in about 80% of cases, and polydactyly and polycystic kidneys are found in many fetuses/infants with trisomy 13. Table 7-4 summarizes the common physical findings in trisomy 13.

> ■ **TABLE 7-4.** Features of Trisomy 13
>
> - Cleft lip and palate
> - Microphthalmia
> - Microcephaly
> - Closely spaced eyes
> - Other eye defects

Case 2: A 30-year-old woman with two first trimester spontaneous abortions presents to you to discuss the chromosome result from her recent loss. That report indicates the finding of trisomy 16.

Chromosome abnormalities are a significant cause of reproductive loss. Of the 15% to 20% of clinical pregnancies that end in miscarriage, between 50% and 75% of them are the result of a chromosome abnormality. Although almost any type of abnormality can be seen in miscarriage material, the most common findings are trisomy 16, trisomy 22, monosomy X, and triploidy.[8] In the second trimester, trisomies 13, 18, 21 along with monosomy X are the common abnormalities found, and explain between 20% and 50% of second trimester losses. In the third trimester the likelihood of finding a chromosomal abnormality as the explanation for a stillbirth is approximately 5%. However, as will be discussed in later chapters, analyzing reproductive losses using microarray or sequencing technologies may markedly increase the incidence of genetic abnormalities as the cause for these losses.

Triploidy represents three complete sets of chromosomes, and can result from two different mechanisms. In diandric conceptions, an egg is fertilized by 2 sperm resulting in 69 chromosomes. In a dygenic triploid conception, an egg with a duplicated set of chromosomes (46) is fertilized by a single sperm (23) resulting in 69 chromosomes. Both forms of triploidy result in very high loss rates in the first trimester, but of those that progress into the second trimester the clinical phenotype varies significantly between those that are diandric and those that are digynic. Diandric pregnancies have a fetus with moderate, relatively symmetric growth restriction, but with a large, cystic placenta. In digynic triploids, the fetus has severe asymmetric growth restriction with a very small noncystic placenta. It should be clear from the clinical presentation of the diandric triploid that this chromosome abnormality is the underlying etiology of most partial molar pregnancies.

The key counseling points to Case 2 are quite straightforward. First, the pregnancy loss was because of a lethal genetic condition, and occurred as a random event prior to conception. Second, there are no known intrinsic or extrinsic factors that result in nondisjunction other than maternal age. Therefore, a "genetic evaluation" of the couple is not necessary. Third, an explanation is known for this loss, and given the high frequency of similar findings in early pregnancy losses, her first loss was likely also a random event. Proceeding with a work-up for recurrent pregnancy loss would not be productive given these findings. Finally, at the current time the majority of geneticists would counsel that the finding of a lethal trisomy in a spontaneous loss would not indicate an increased risk for a subsequent trisomic conception. However, research presently underway could find that there are genetic determinants that result in some individuals having a greater likelihood of nondisjunction, and therefore a greater likelihood of a trisomic offspring. It is incumbent upon the practicing physician to stay current in this area in order to provide appropriate reproductive counseling.

Case 3: Your 28-year-old patient in her first pregnancy was found to have a fetal cystic hygroma on an ultrasound performed at 18 weeks' gestation. A subsequent amniocentesis revealed a karyotype of 45,X. How would you counsel the patient.

Turner syndrome occurs in approximately 1 in every 2500 live births, but is much more common in early pregnancies.[2] It is thought that more than 90% of 45,X conceptions end in spontaneous loss, and, as noted previously, it is a common finding in spontaneous abortions. In the second trimester it may present with a cystic hygroma with, or without, fetal hydrops.

Infants with Turner syndrome (TS) commonly have a short neck with a webbed appearance, puffy hands and feet, and a low hairline. All of these features are thought to be secondary to the effects of the previously present cystic hygroma and anasarca. The major issues for children and young adults with TS are short stature (average height is 4 ft 8 in) and ovarian failure. Most girls with TS experience ovarian failure early in childhood, and thus do not enter puberty. However, some individuals may have some breast development, normal menses, and ovarian failure in late teens or early twenties. Cardiac malformations, specifically coarctation of the aorta, occur in approximately 10% of TS patients, and up to a third will have some form of renal malformation.

Individuals with TS have normal intelligence and verbal skills are likewise normal. However, some girls with TS have difficulty with visual-spatial tasks and with learning math which has been called the "Turner neurocognitive phenotype."

The key counseling points for this patient revolve around providing the family with clear expectations about the clinical features associated with TS, and the available treatment options. Second, recommending a fetal echocardiogram to assess for coarctation of the aorta is essential for providing complete prognostic information.

■ CONCLUSION

Having a basic understanding of common chromosome problems is an essential skill set for the practicing obstetrician-gynecologist. In addition to those abnormalities discussed in this chapter, Chapter 14 on infertility and pregnancy loss contains additional information on Turner syndrome, and a summary of the features of Klinefelter syndrome.

REFERENCES

1. Lejeune J, Turpin R, Gautier M. Chromosomic diagnosis of mongolism. *Arch Fr Pediatr.* 1959;16:962-963.

2. Jones KL. *Smith's Recognizable Patterns of Human Malformations.* 6th ed. Philadelphia, PA: Elsevier Saunders; 2006.

3. Hook EB, Cross PK, Schreinemachers DM. Chromosomal abnormality rates at amniocentesis and in live-born infants. *JAMA.* 1983;249:2034-2038.

4. Cross PK, Hook EB. Rates of trisomies 21, 18, 12 and other chromosome abnormalities in about 20,000 prenatal studies compared with estimated rates in live births. *Hum Genet.* 1982;61:318-324.

5. Stern J. Detection of higher recurrence risk for age-dependent chromosome abnormalities with an application to trisomy G1. (Down's syndrome) *Hum Hered.* 1970;20:112-122.

6. Morris JK, Mutton DE, Alberman E. Recurrences of free trisomy 21. Analysis of data from the National Down Syndrome Cytogenetics Register. *Prenatal Diagn.* 2005;25:1120-1128.

7. Bugge M, Collins A, Peterson MB, et al. Non-disjunction of chromosome 18. *Hum Mol Genet.* 1998;7:661-669.

8. Gardner RJM, Sutherland GR, Shaffer LG. *Chromosome Abnormalities and Genetic Counseling.* Oxford: Oxford University Press; 2012.

Screening for Genetic Disorders in Pregnancy

Case 1: A 25-year-old Caucasian (Northern European ancestry) G_1 presents for her first prenatal visit at 10 weeks' gestation. Her medical and family history is negative for any factors that are of concern for this pregnancy.

The phrase "screening for genetic disorders" generally refers to two forms of genetic testing. One approach is screening the patient and/or spouse to determine their carrier status for common genetic disorders, such as cystic fibrosis. Secondly, the genetic screening may refer to techniques that assess the likelihood the fetus is affected by a genetic condition or birth defect, such as Down syndrome (DS) or spina bifida. Although both are termed "screening," the concepts behind each approach are significantly different.

■ CARRIER SCREENING

Screening for carrier status can either be directed to certain high-risk groups, or can be population based. Carrier screening for specific ethnic groups has been covered in Chapter 6 on *Preconception Counseling*. The approaches described previously for the patient contemplating a pregnancy are the same ones used for the pregnant patient. However, depending on the patient's gestational age, concurrent testing of the patient and her spouse may be necessary to provide adequate time for prenatal diagnosis, should both parents be found to be carriers of the genetic condition in question.

Population based screening, on the other hand, means that every pregnant woman, regardless of her ethnic background, is offered carrier screening. At the time of the writing of this book, only cystic fibrosis falls in this category. Although more common in individuals with northern European heritage, the mutant gene is found in all populations. This factor and the pluralistic nature of US society has lead the American College of Obstetricians and Gynecologists (ACOG) to suggest that all women should be offered carrier screening for cystic fibrosis.[1] One drawback to the current recommendation is that the recommended panel of mutations that should be tested for is based on the most common mutations in the "Caucasian" population, and may, therefore, detect very few carriers in an Asian populations.

In all forms of genetic screening, but especially in carrier screening, both the patient and the physician need to be well versed in the benefits and limitations of the testing. Using our Caucasian patient example, we know that the incidence of CF carriers in this population is 1 in 29. There are nearly 2000 mutations that have been found to cause cystic fibrosis, but testing for the 23 common mutations will detect approximately 90% of the carriers. If the patient is negative for the common CF mutations, her chances of having a child with CF are quite low, but it is not zero. Should she be found to carry a CF mutation, and her spouse have negative testing, their risk of having an affected child is approximately one in a thousand. Although a low risk, it is significantly higher than the population incidence of CF (1 in 3000 births).

The key points in counseling the patient about carrier screening is that she should be provided information on the clinical features and natural history of the disorder, the benefits and limitations of the testing, and the options available to her, should she and her spouse both be carriers of the genetic condition. For any new genetic disorder to be introduced on a population-wide basis, the carrier frequency should be significantly high (eg, the 1 in 29 incidence of CF) and be comparably high in all ethnic groups. Likewise, the screening test itself must be relatively inexpensive, detect most of the carriers (ideally 95% or greater), and the test results must be easily interpretable by the practicing physician.

> **Case 2: Ms. Canick is a 30-year-old G_3P_2 who is now 8 weeks' gestation. She had a "triple" screen in her previous pregnancies, and wants to know whether there are earlier and better options to determine if she is carrying a Down syndrome fetus. What options do you discuss with her?**

■ SCREENING FOR FETAL GENETIC CONDITIONS

Screening has been defined as "the identification, among apparently healthy individuals, of those who are sufficiently at risk for a specific disorder to justify a

■ **TABLE 8-1.** Down Syndrome Screening Tests and Detection Rates	
Screen Test Rate (%)	**Detection**
First Trimester	
NT measurement	60
NT measurement, PAPP-A, free or total β-hCG	85
Second Trimester	
Triple screen (MSAFP, hCG, unconjugated estriol)	60
Quadruple screen (MSAFP, hCG, unconjugated estriol, inhibin A)	80
First Plus Second Trimester	
Integrated (NT, PAPP-A, quad screen)	95
Stepwise sequential	95
First-trimester test offered	
Positive: diagnostic test offered	
Negative: second-trimester test offered	
Final: risk assessment incorporates first and second results	
Contingent sequential	95
First-trimester test result:	
Positive: diagnostic test offered	
Negative: no further testing	
Intermediate: second-trimester test offered	
Final: risk assessment incorporates first and second results	

Abbreviations: hCG, human chorionic gonadotropin; MSAFP, maternal serum alpha-fetoprotein; NT, nuchal translucency; PAPP-A, pregnancy-associated plasma protein A; quad, quadruple.

subsequent diagnostic test or procedure."[2] It can be said that the first screening test for genetic disease in the fetus was the use of the patient's birth date to determine the at-risk category for pregnancies complicated by a fetal chromosomal disorder. When introduced as a criterion for offering amniocentesis, the screen positive rate would have been 5% (the percent of pregnant women age 35 or greater in the US population in the early 1970s) with a detection rate of approximately 30% (the number of DS children born to women above the age of 35). It is important to note here that screening for genetic diseases in pregnancy has not followed the conventional screening terminology of sensitivity, specificity, false positive, and false negative. Even when using the term "false positive" the author most commonly is actually describing the "screen positive" rate. Screen positive refers to the number of individuals in the population who have a positive screening test, and includes both the true positives and the false positives. Because the incidence of true positives is quite low, the screen positive and false positive rates are essentially the same, and used interchangeably by most authors. Pregnancy screening programs use a second measure, known as detection rate (the percentage of true positives that are found using the screening algorithm), which is synonymous with sensitivity. To put our maternal age example into a current context the screen positive rate would be 15% to 20% (the percentage of US pregnancies in women aged 35 or older) for a similar detection rate of between 30% and 40% for DS. By any measure, this approach to screening would have no validity. Since the early 1980s, there have been many attempts to define serum and ultrasound markers that would more accurately delineate the at-risk population for DS, as well as other birth defects. This chapter will focus on three of these approaches for DS screening to outline the principles, as well as the benefits and limitations, of screening.

Multiple Marker Screening

The most commonly used second-trimester screen is called the quadruple (quad) screen because it uses four biochemical measures—human chorionic gonadotropin (hCG), unconjugated estriol (uE$_3$), inhibin A, and alpha-fetoprotein (AFP) in combination with the patient's age to generate a risk that the fetus has DS. DS pregnancies are associated with higher levels of hCG and inhibin A, and lower levels of AFP and uE$_3$ than chromosomally normal pregnancies. By using these analyte measurements to create a series of likelihood ratios, and combining that information with the patient's age-related risk, each patient can be provided with a specific risk for her pregnancy. In the United States a "positive" test result has been defined as a risk of having a child with DS that is greater than or equal to that of a 35-year-old (1 in 270). Using this cut-off the screen positive rate in the overall US population will be approximately 5% with a DS detection rate of 80%. Quad screening will detect a similar percentage of trisomy 18 pregnancies, but will detect very few, if any, trisomy 13 fetuses, or fetuses with sex chromosome aneuploidy.[3]

There are several key issues in both pretest and posttest counseling for quad screening that should be part of the discussion with pregnant patients. First, as noted above, the screen is only good for the detection of trisomy 21 and trisomy 18, and one in five of these pregnancies will be missed by quad screening. Second, a screen positive result is almost always a false positive result, and no action should be undertaken until amniocentesis has confirmed a positive result. Third, when the patient has a result in hand (eg, a 1 in 50 risk for DS), the population information is no longer useful to providing counseling. She should be provided the information that 1 in 50 women with her result will be carrying a DS fetus, and 49 out of 50 will not. This result is in effect indicating for her personally a 98% "false positive" rate. Providing balanced, nondirective counseling allows the patient to make an informed decision about whether amniocentesis is appropriate for her.

First-Trimester Screening

Early studies on screening for DS in the first trimester proceeded on two parallel pathways: serum markers and ultrasound markers. Initial serum marker studies using hCG (elevated in DS) and pregnancy-associated plasma protein A (PAPP-A) which is low in DS pregnancies yielded a detection rate of 60% with a screen positive rate of 5%.[4] At the same time the ultrasound community had discovered that an increased amount of fluid at the back of the fetal neck (referred to as nuchal translucency) was associated with fetal chromosomal abnormalities. Early studies in high-risk populations found that detection rates of 80% or greater were possible for trisomy 21, 18, and 13.[5] On the other hand, nuchal translucency (NT) measurements in low-risk populations had detection rates that were closer to the 60% seen in serum testing alone. However, combining serum markers with NT measurements, and the patient's age, provided a screening tool that could detect approximately 85% of DS pregnancies with a 5% positive screening rate.[3,4] In addition to the slightly better detection rate with the first-trimester combined test, the patient has the option for early information, whether that be reassuring in low-risk circumstances, or the ability for an early diagnosis by CVS in cases with high-risk screening results.

There are several variations on the combined use of both first- and second-trimester screening. One approach is the integrated test, which uses the NT measurement and PAPP-A from a first-trimester visit with a second-trimester quad screen, and reports a second-trimester risk based on these six markers. No information is provided to the patient at the time of the first-trimester testing. The benefit is a detection rate of approximately 95%, but with the limitation that the results are available only in the second trimester.[6] Alternatives to this approach are the stepwise sequential test and the contingent test. In the stepwise sequential a positive result in the first trimester is acted upon. A patient with a negative first-trimester screen then has a quad screen, but it takes into account the risk from the first-trimester screen to create the new risk. The quad screen must use the patient's risk figure from the first-trimester screen, not the patient's age related risk. It would be expected to detect 95% of DS pregnancies, but is logistically complicated to administer to a large population. In contingent screening, first-trimester results are categorized as high risk, low risk, and intermediate risk. Those with high risk (1 in 50) are offered CVS. Those with low risk (1 in 1500) have no further testing. Those with intermediate risks have a quad screen done and follow the algorithm for second-trimester screening. Like stepwise sequential screening, the detection rate approaches 95%, but the administrative difficulties of getting the intermediate group to return for the quad screen can be significant.[7] It is essential that the patient not have both a first-trimester screen and a second-trimester screen done independently of one of these algorithms. When done as independent tests the detection rate will be high, but the false positive rate will be 10% or more. Table 8-1 summarizes the detection rates of the various screening modalities assuming a 5% false positive rate.

Noninvasive Prenatal Testing

Noninvasive prenatal testing (NTPT) refers to using cell-free fetal DNA circulating in the maternal circulation. This cell-free fetal DNA appears to be derived from the placenta and comprises between 3% and 13% of total cell-free maternal DNA. Using powerful genomic tools, such as massively parallel genomic sequencing (Figure 8-1), many groups have been accurately detecting the common trisomies

General Principle of Noninvasive Detection of Trisomy 21 by Shotgun Sequencing

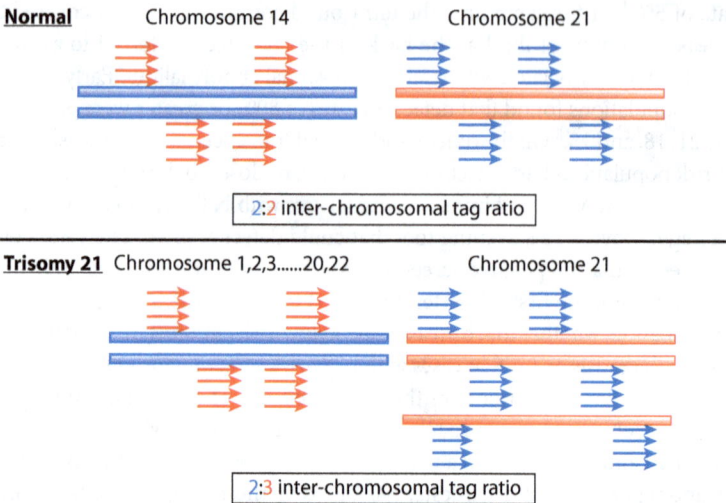

FIGURE 8-1. By analyzing multiple segments of chromosome 21 compared to another chromosome, such as 14, a change in ratio from the normal 2:2 to the 2:3 in Down syndrome can be detected.

as well as sex chromosome aneuploidies.[8–11] In high-risk populations the detection rates for trisomy 21 and 18 have been approximately 99% with false positive rates of less than 0.5%. Detection rates for trisomy 13, and sex chromosome aneuploidies have been somewhat lower. In these studies the false positives are true false positives, and likely represent aneuploidy present in the placenta, but not in the fetus. In low risk populations, the proportion of patients with the positive test that carry affected child (positive predictive value) for NIPT is approximately 45% for Trisomy 21 and 40% for Trisomy 18 as compared to 4.2% for Trisomy 21 and 8.3% for Trisomy 18 in the First Trimester screening. The negative predictive value for NIPT is 99.8% and 98% for First trimester screening. DNA-based screening ultimately will replace both serum and ultrasound markers for aneuploidy screening. However, despite its high sensitivity in the detection of aneuploidy, patients will need to be counseled that it does not have the diagnostic accuracy of either amniocentesis or CVS. Although the false positive rate is low at approximately 0.5%, patients must be cautioned that a diagnostic test must be performed before making any decision regarding pregnancy termination. The source of the free fetal DNA appears to be trophoblast, and it is well known from CVS testing that chromosome abnormalities, such as trisomy 18, can be found in the placental (placental mosaicism) that are not present in the fetus. It should not be surprising that a recent report described eight cases of false positive results for both trisomy 18 and trisomy 13.[12]

■ CONCLUSION

In the nearly 50 years since the era of prenatal diagnosis began, the pace of innovation has been astounding. However, the overall concepts remain unchanged. Testing should be offered to women who, after being fully informed of the benefits and limitations of the testing, desire to have more knowledge about the genetic status of their fetuses.

REFERENCES

1. American College of Obstetricians and Gynecologists Committee on Genetics. ACOG Committee Opinion No. 486: update on carrier screening for cystic fibrosis. *Obstet Gynecol.* 2011;117(4):1028-1031.

2. Cuckle HS, Wald NJ. Principles of screening. In: Wald NJ, ed. *Antenatal and Neonatal Screening,* Oxford: Oxford University Press; 1984:1-22.

3. Malone FD, Canick JA, Ball RH, et al. First-trimester or second-trimester screening, or both, for Down's syndrome. *N Engl J Med.* 2005;353:2001-2011.

4. Wald NJ, Hackshaw AK. Combining ultrasound and biochemistry in first-trimester screening for Down's syndrome. *Prenat Diagn.* 1997;17:821-829.

5. Snijders RL, Noble P, Sebire N, et al. UK multicenter project on assessment of risk of trisomy 21 by maternal age and fetal nuchal-translucency thickness at 10-14 weeks of gestation. *Lancet.* 1998;352:343-346.

6. Wald NJ, Watt HC, Hackshaw AK. Integrated screening for Down's syndrome on the basis of tests performed during the first and second trimester. *N Engl J Med.* 1999;341:461-467.

7. Cuckle HS, Malone FD, Wright D. Contingent screening for Down syndrome—results from the FaSTER trial. *Prenat Diagn.* 2008;28(2):89-94.

8. Palomaki GE, Deciu C, Kloza EM, et al. DNA sequencing of maternal plasma reliably identifies trisomy 18 and trisomy 13 as well as Down syndrome: an international collaborative study. *Genet Med.* 2012;14:296-305.

9. Bianchi DW, Platt LD, Goldberg JD, et al. Genome-wide fetal aneuploidy detection by maternal plasma DNA sequencing. *Obstet Gynecol.* 2012;119:890-901.

10. Norton ME, Brar H, Weiss J, et al. Non-invasive chromosomal evaluation (NICE) study: results of a multicenter, prospective, cohort study for detection of fetal trisomy 18. *Am J Obstet Gynecol.* 2012;207(2):137.e1-137.e8.

11. Nicolaides KH, Syngelaki A, Ashoor G, et al. Noninvasive prenatal testing for fetal trisomies in a routinely screened first-trimester population. *Am J Obstet Gynecol.* 2012;207:374.e1-374.e6.

12. Mennuti MT, Cherry AM, Morrissette JJD, Dugoff L. Is it time to sound an alarm about false-positive cell-free DNA testing for fetal aneuploidy? *Am J Obstet Gynecol.* 2013 Mar 22. Pii:S0002-9378(13)00301-3. doi:10.1016/j.ajog.2013.03.027.

Methods of Prenatal Diagnosis

CHAPTER 9

- **DIAGNOSTIC TESTING**
  Amniocentesis
  Chorionic Villus Sampling
  Ultrasound
  Preimplantation Genetic Diagnosis
- **CONCLUSION**

Case 1: A 35-year-old, gravida 1, presents for prenatal care at 8 weeks' gestation. How do you counsel her regarding her risks for genetic conditions in her fetus, and her options for prenatal screening and/or diagnosis?

Historically prenatal diagnosis was offered to all women who would be age 35 or greater at delivery. The exact reason that age 35 was chosen in the United States (in the United Kingdom age 37 was chosen) is not entirely clear, but it was not because there is a biological difference between women above, and those below, age 35 that causes a sudden increase in the risk of chromosome abnormalities in their offspring. Likewise, the age cut-off was not chosen to balance the risk of a chromosomal abnormality with the risk of procedure-related pregnancy loss, as the guidelines were established before the early studies were done to assess procedure related risk. The best explanations are those based on logistics: what resources were available to provide cytogenetic studies to the population of women. In the early 1970s when amniocentesis was introduced into practice the limited number of cytogenetic laboratories available in the United States could provide testing for about 5% of the pregnant population. At that time only 5% of the pregnant population was 35 or older at birth. Whatever the actual reason for defining age 35 or greater as "advanced maternal age," it became the US standard of care until 2007 when the American College of Obstetricians and Gynecologists (ACOG) declared that age 35 should no longer be used as a criteria for whether a patient should be offered invasive prenatal testing.[1]

Although the risk of chromosomal abnormalities such as Down syndrome (DS) does increase with maternal age, using maternal age as a screening criterion results in a very poor screening testing. With approximately 15% of the US population age 35 or older, there would be a 15% "false positive" rate to detect about 30% of DS fetuses. In 1975, when no other screening methods were available, a 5% false positive with a 30% detection was a more reasonable approach.

In counseling the patient described above, it is important to present the risk in terms that are understandable to the patient. Table 9-1 presents the risks of DS and all chromosomal abnormalities at both mid-trimester and at birth. At age 35 the mid-trimester risk (the standard time for most testing) of DS is 1/270, and for all chromosomal abnormalities 1/100. Giving these numbers as fractions or percentages (0.3% and 1%) is not truly understood by most patients. Putting these numbers in concrete terms, such as "1 in every 100 women of your age will have a chromosome abnormality in their pregnancy," is more likely to convey the information in a way to allow an informed decision. The counseling session should include some discussion of the natural history of the disorders that are included in the category of "all chromosomal abnormalities." By the late first and early second trimester, only five maternal age-associated chromosome aneuploidies are likely to be present in a viable pregnancy (trisomies 13, 18, and 21, and the sex chromosome aneuploidies, 47,XXY and 47,XXX). Turner syndrome (45,X) is not associated with advancing maternal age. Finally, the counseling session should emphasize that increasing maternal age is only associated with a risk of nondisjunction (chromosome abnormalities), and not with any other genetic conditions. Having provided to the patient this brief discussion of her risks, attention can be turned to the various diagnostic and screening options available to her. It is

■ **TABLE 9-1.** Age-Related Risk of Trisomy 21 and all Chromosome Abnormalities

| Age | Trisomy 21 | | All Chromosomes | |
	Mid-pregnancy	Birth	Mid-pregnancy	Birth
33	1/450	1/600	1/200	1/300
34	1/350	1/400	1/200	1/250
35	1/270	1/380	1/100	1/200
36	1/210	1/290	1/100	1/170
37	1/166	1/230	1/75	1/140
38	1/129	1/180	1/75	1/110
39	1/100	1/140	1/50	1/90
40	1/78	1/110	1/50	1/70
41	1/60	1/80	1/30	1/60
42	1/45	1/65	1/30	1/50
43	1/35	1/50	1/20	1/40
44	1/30	1/40	1/20	1/30
45	1/20	1/30	1/13	1/20
46	1/17	1/25	1/13	1/20

important to remember that "doing nothing" also is an appropriate option, given the 99% likelihood that the pregnancy is not complicated by DS, or one of the other aneuploidies.

◼ DIAGNOSTIC TESTING

Amniocentesis

The "gold standard" in prenatal diagnosis is amniocentesis, having now been a part of the medical practice for nearly 50 years. It is generally performed between 16 and 18 weeks' gestation for genetic diagnosis, but can be performed at later gestational ages, if clinically indicated. Studies of amniocentesis done prior to 14 weeks' gestation have found higher fetal loss rates (corrected for earlier gestational age), and an increased incidence of positional limb abnormalities, such as club foot. Current indications for offering amniocentesis, which are also the indications for prenatal diagnosis in general, are outlined in Table 9-2.

In counseling a patient regarding the risks and benefits of amniocentesis, the greatest benefit is quite precise genetic information, approaching 100% reliability for the common indications for amniocentesis. The most common reason for a misdiagnosis is contamination of the amniotic fluid sample by maternal cells obtained as the needle passes through maternal tissue before entering the amniotic cavity. This risk can be minimized by discarding the first 1 to 2 mL of amniotic fluid withdrawn, which should clear the needle tip of any potential maternal tissue.

The most significant risk of amniocentesis is procedure-related fetal loss. Despite nearly a half century since its introduction, the true risk of fetal loss directly related to amniocentesis remains unknown. The first US study funded by the National Institute of Health found that the overall fetal loss rate was 3.5% compared to a 3.2% loss rate in the control group, a difference that was not statistically significant.[2] Despite this lack of statistical significance, a number of textbooks begin stating that the risk of amniocentesis was 0.5% or less, which ultimately became "the risk of spontaneous abortion following amniocentesis is one in 200." The only randomized study of the risk of amniocentesis, performed by Tabor and colleagues did find a statistically significant risk of pregnancy loss following amniocentesis of approximately 1%.[3] Since this study from the mid-1980s a number of observational studies have been published, each failing to find a significant

---

◼ **TABLE 9-2.** Indications for Amniocentesis

- Previous child with autosomal trisomy
- Either parent is a carrier of a chromosomal rearrangement
- Previous child, patient or spouse with a neural tube defect
- Abnormal maternal serum markers
- Abnormal first trimester screen
- Pregnancy at risk for diagnosable genetic disorder
- Ultrasound findings

difference in pregnancy loss in patients undergoing amniocentesis.[4,5] However, each study has consistently shown a higher, albeit not statistically significant, risk for the amniocentesis group compared to the control groups. For purpose of counseling a patient considering amniocentesis, the best approach may be to state that the risk of pregnancy loss following amniocentesis is quite low, likely in the range of 1 loss for every 500 to 1000 procedures performed. If the procedure is performed by an experienced operator using continuous ultrasound guidance, there should be no other maternal or fetal risks associated with amniocentesis.

Chorionic Villus Sampling

Chorionic villus sampling (CVS) was introduced into Western medicine in the early 1980s as an alternative to amniocentesis that could be performed in the first trimester of pregnancy.[6] Although the concept of using a plastic catheter introduced through the cervix to aspirate placental villi had been put forward by Chinese investigators a decade earlier, consistent success in obtaining villi only occurred with the introduction of real-time ultrasound technology. Ultrasound provided the ability to locate the exact placental location, and to provide continuous observation of the catheter to allow precise placement and thus successful sampling of villus material. Later transabdominal CVS was introduced using a needle to aspirate villi from placental locations that previously had been difficult or impossible to reach by a transcervically placed catheter.

There were two early studies, one from the United States and one from Canada, comparing the risk of CVS to that of amniocentesis. Both studies were consistent, indicating an approximately 1% greater loss in the CVS group compared to the amniocentesis group.[6,7] Assuming that the risk of amniocentesis was 0.5%, textbooks began quoting a risk of spontaneous loss from CVS to be 1.5%. Subsequently, a number of observational studies have been completed which suggest the increased risks seen in the early studies reflect lack of experience of the operators, not an intrinsically greater risk of CVS.[8,9] Currently, most agree that in experienced centers the risk of procedure-related loss is the same for both CVS and amniocentesis.[10] However, in counseling patients it is important to emphasize the significantly greater background loss rate in the first trimester, when CVS is performed, compared to the second trimester, when amniocentesis is performed.

The early studies of CVS were done using procedure times of 9 to 12 6/7 weeks' gestation; therefore no information was obtained on the risks of transcervical CVS after the first trimester. Later studies comparing CVS to early amniocentesis were performed using transabdominal CVS only. Given this lack of safety data, many operators perform transcervical CVS from 10 to 12 6/7 weeks' gestation, and use the transabdominal approach if CVS is necessary at 13 weeks or greater.

The change in timing of CVS from 9 gestational weeks to 10, occurred following reports of an increased risk of birth defects, specifically transverse limb abnormalities, following CVS at very early gestational ages (5-8 weeks).[11,12] Importantly, studies of CVS done after 10 weeks' gestation have shown no increased risk in the incidence of any birth defects.[13,14]

> ■ **TABLE 9-3.** Indications for CVS
>
> - Previous child with autosomal trisomy
> - Either parent is a carrier of a chromosomal rearrangement
> - Abnormal first trimester screen
> - Pregnancy at risk for diagnosable genetic disorder
> - Ultrasound findings

CVS has one other "complication" that is uniquely different from amniocentesis. In approximately 1% to 2% of CVS samples two cell lines (one normal, one abnormal) will be found. Approximately 10% to 25% of the cases will reflect true chromosome mosaicism in the fetus. The remaining 75% to 90% will be mosaicism that is "confined" to the placenta. This "complication" of CVS directly lead to the understanding of embryo rescue and uniparental disomy that is discussed in more detail in Chapter 2. However, because of placental mosaicism, approximately 1 in 100 patients undergoing CVS will need to have a follow-up amniocentesis to determine the true fetal status.

The indications for CVS are depicted in Table 9-3, and they are quite comparable to those of amniocentesis. Obviously, an abnormal second-trimester screen is not an indication for CVS. Likewise, because testing for alpha-fetoprotein requires an amniotic fluid sample, CVS is not indicated for the pregnancy at risk for a neural tube defect.

> **Case 2: Ms. Edwards is a 26-year-old whose first pregnancy was complicated by the finding of bilateral club feet in her fetus. Chromosome studies and microarray testing were negative. After birth her child was evaluated by a clinical geneticist, and she was told that it was an isolated birth defect. She is now 12 weeks' pregnant, and would like to know what the chance is of having another child with club feet, and what testing she should have in this pregnancy.**

Ultrasound

Although ultrasound is most commonly used in low-risk pregnancies as a screening tool, there are many circumstances when it is a prenatal diagnostic tool. In a circumstance where a pregnancy is known to be at risk for X-linked hydrocephalus, the ultrasound finding of ventriculomegaly is "diagnostic" of recurrence. On the other hand, the absence of ventriculomegaly on a mid-trimester scan may not be diagnostic of an unaffected pregnancy, if the natural history includes a later onset of enlarged ventricles.

When a screening ultrasound "diagnoses" a birth defect, such as a congenital heart defect, the scan may be diagnostic for the type of heart defect, but not the etiology of the heart defect. The job of the prenatal diagnostician is to recommend the necessary additional testing to determine if the defect is isolated, or is part of a specific genetic syndrome. For this reason there are very few instances in which ultrasound should be considered diagnostic. It is generally the first step in a comprehensive diagnostic evaluation that may include further imaging studies and invasive testing, such as amniocentesis.

The counseling for Ms. Edwards is that isolated club feet is a multifactorial condition (see Chapter 3), and has an approximately 3% risk of occurring in this pregnancy. Neither CVS nor amniocentesis would be useful in the current pregnancy because the genetic evaluation was negative in the previous pregnancy. She should be offered a detailed ultrasound evaluation at 18 to 20 weeks' gestation, which would be "diagnostic" as either the presence, or absence, of clubbing should be detected by a skilled sonologist.

> **Case 3: Ms. Sachs is a 28-year-old of Ashkenazi Jewish ancestry. She and her spouse are carriers of the Canavan gene mutation. Each has a different mutation, but each mutation is one of the common mutations in their ethnic group. In her two previous pregnancies, she had CVS for mutation testing, and both fetuses were affected. She elected to terminate those pregnancies. Currently she is not pregnant, and wants to discuss the option of pre-implantation genetic diagnosis to prevent having to terminate another pregnancy.**

Preimplantation Genetic Diagnosis

Preimplantation genetic diagnosis (PGD) is used to describe genetic testing that occurs before an embryo implants in the uterus. There are three approaches that have been utilized.[15] First, the polar body can be removed, and the genetic status of the oocyte inferred from the results of the polar body assay.[16] In the circumstance where the polar body has the mutated gene, the oocyte is inferred to be "normal," and therefore an embryo obtained by fertilization of this oocyte would be unaffected with the genetic condition of interest. A second method of PGD is blastomere biopsy; one or two blastomeres are removed from an eight-cell embryo, and analyzed for the genetic condition of interest. Only embryos found not to have the genetic mutation are transferred into the uterus. This is the method that has been most commonly used to-date.[17] Finally, PGD can be performed at the blastocyst stage by sampling a portion of the trophectoderm (early placenta) by a trophectoderm biopsy. All three approaches appear to be safe, with studies done to-date showing no increased risk of birth defects or growth disorders in infants born after PGD when compared to infants born after other assisted reproductive technologies.[18]

Each technique is associated with some limitations. Polar body testing can result in an erroneous diagnosis because of crossing over occurring during meiosis. This limitation has become rare as newer technologies of direct gene testing have been introduced, compared to earlier studies that used markers that were closely linked to the gene. However, its major limitation for recessive disorders is that polar body biopsy only determines the maternal contributions to the embryo.

■ TABLE 9-4. Common Mendelian disorders for which PGD is offered:	
Most Common	**Less Common**
Thalassemias	Charcot-Marie-Tooth
Cystic Fibrosis	Adenomatosis Polyposis Coli (APC)
Huntington Disease	Epidermolysis bullosa
Myotonic Dystrophy	Fanconi Anemia
Rh	Fragile X
Sickle Cell Anemia	Gaucher disease
Spinal Muscular Atrophy	Marfan syndrome
Tay Sachs Disease	Osteogenesis imperfecta (AD)
	Sanhoff disease

A finding that the embryo will have the maternal mutation does not differentiate between a carrier and an affected embryo; thus decreasing the number of embryos that are "unaffected" to only those that receive the normal allele from the mother. Blastomere biopsy is subject to error for two reasons related to the requirement to amplify the DNA from a single cell by the polymerase chain reaction. Residual sperm present in zona pellucida can be a source of DNA contamination resulting in amplifying the paternal, and not the fetal DNA. However, current molecular technologies using single nucleotide polymorphisms and short tandem repeats allow simultaneous mutation detection and marker analysis, almost completely eliminating the risk of misdiagnosis by sperm contamination. When testing for a recessive disease where each parent carries a different mutation, failure to amplify one of the mutations (allele dropout) results in a misdiagnosis of a carrier embryo, rather than the true diagnosis of an affected embryo. As with sperm contamination, newer molecular techniques, such as microarrays with whole genome amplification will provide methods to overcome this problem as well. Blastocyst biopsy has the benefit of providing more cells, but requires a longer culture period. Because of the late stage when the biopsy is done, any genetic testing must be done rapidly, within 24 hours, or the biopsied blastocysts must be cryopreserved for later use. Table 9-4 lists some of the disorders for which PGD may be appropriate.

In the mid-1990s, the use of fluorescence in situ hybridization (FISH) with chromosome-specific probes were introduced, and applied to single cell biopsies from preimplantation embryos.[19] The hope was that by detecting aneuploid embryos in women of older age, and those with recurrent pregnancy loss that the IVF pregnancy rates could be improved. One of the first problems noted was the high incidence of mosaicism for chromosome aneuploidy in tested embryos. In many cases, the test result (abnormal or normal) reflected only a minority of the cells in the overall embryo. At the same time, a large randomized trial of the use of what has been termed preimplantation genetic screening (PGS) found that live-birth rates were significantly decreased in women having PGS.[20] Therefore, the benefits of PGS to improve IVF pregnancy rates in women of older age, or those with recurrent pregnancy loss, remain the subject of intense debate. It is hoped that the use of blastocyst biopsies with microarray-based genomewide chromosome screening, instead of only assaying for eight chromosomes by FISH, will prove to be a beneficial approach to these difficult clinical issues.[21]

Ms. Sachs' case emphasizes the issue of "probabilities." Although she has only a 25% risk of having an affected pregnancy, both of her pregnancies have been affected. Despite having two affected pregnancies, she still has the same 25% risk of recurrence in the next pregnancy. However, the emotional stress of having to terminate another pregnancy may be overwhelming for some couples. PGD offers the possibility for an unaffected pregnancy, but with the significant limitation that it requires *in vitro* fertilization with its attendant risks and costs. Ms. Sachs would benefit from an extensive counseling session with a geneticist versed in all prenatal and preimplantation diagnostic options.

■ CONCLUSION

In summary, prenatal diagnostic procedures continue to play a significant role in the prenatal detection of genetic disorders. In experienced centers, they provide a safe, and highly accurate approach to assessing fetal status. Although the advent of more precise screening protocols helps to focus their utilization on the highest risk population, newer molecular techniques that offer concurrent detection of multiple genetic disorders through whole genome sequencing may lead to a marked increase in the utilization of diagnostic procedures because of their ability to provide an adequate sample for this multiplex testing.

REFERENCES

1. ACOG Committee on Practice Bulletins, ACOG Practice Bulletin No. 77. Screening for fetal chromosomal abnormalities. *Obstet Gynecol.* 2007;109:217-227.

2. The NICHD National Registry for Amniocentesis Study Group. Midtrimester amniocentesis for prenatal diagnosis. *JAMA.* 1976;236:1471-1476.

3. Tabor A, Philip J, Madsen M, et al. Randomised controlled trial of genetic amniocentesis in 4606 low-risk women. *Lancet.* 1986;1:1287-1293.

4. Eddleman KA, Malone FD, Sullivan L, et al. Pregnancy loss rates after midtrimester amniocentesis. *Obstet Gynecol.* 2006;109:1067-1072.

5. Odibo AO, Gray DL, Dicke JM, et al. Revisiting the fetal loss rate after second trimester genetic amniocentesis: a single center's 16-year experience. *Obstet Gynecol.* 2008;111:589-595.

6. Rhoads GG, Jackson LG, Schlesselman SE, et al. The safety and efficacy of chorionic villus sampling for early prenatal diagnosis of cytogenetic abnormalities. *N Engl J Med.* 1989;320:609-617.

7. Multicentre randomized clinical trial of chorionic villus sampling and amniocentesis. First report. Canadian Collaborative CVS Amniocentesis Trial Group. *Lancet.* 1989;1:1-6.

8. Caughey AB, Hopkins LM, Norton ME. Chorionic villus sampling compared with amniocentesis and the difference in the rate of pregnancy loss. *Obstet Gynecol.* 2006;108:612-616.

9. Chueh JT, Goldberg JD, Wohlferd MM, Golbus MS. Comparison of transcervical and transabdominal chorionic villus sampling loss rates in nine thousand cases from a single center. *Am J Obstet Gynecol.* 1995;173:1277-1282.

10. Evans MI, Wapner RJ. Invasive prenatal diagnostic procedures 2005. *Semin Perinatol.* 2005;29:215-218.

11. Firth HV, Boyd PA, Chamberlain P, et al. Severe limb abnormalities after chorion villus sampling at 56-66 days' gestation. *Lancet.* 1991;227:762-763.

12. Burton BK, Schulz CJ, Burd LI. Limb anomalies associated with chorionic villus sampling. *Obstet Gynecol.* 1992;79:726-730.

13. Froster UG, Jackson L. Limb defects and chorionic villus sampling results from an international registry, 1992-1994. *Lancet.* 1996;347:489-494.

14. Kuliev A, Jackson L, Froster U, et al. Chorionic villus sampling safety. Report of World Health Organization/EURO meeting in association with the Seventh International Conference on Early Prenatal Diagnosis of Genetic Disease, Tel-Aviv, Israel, May 21, 1994. *Am J Obstet Gynecol.* 1996;174:807-811.

15. Xu K, Montag M. New perspectives on embryo biopsy: not how, but when, and why? *Semin Reprod Med.* 2012;30:259-266.

16. Kuliev A, Rechitsky S. Polar body-based preimplantation genetic diagnosis for Mendelian disorders [review]. *Mol Hum Reprod.* 2011;17:275-285.

17. Harper JC, Wilton L, Traeger-Synodinos J, et al. The ESHRE PGD Consortium: 10 years of data collection. *Hum Reprod Update.* 2012;18(3):234-247.

18. Liebaers I, Desmyttere S, Verpoest W, et al. Report on a consecutive series of 581 children born after blastomere biopsy for preimplantation genetic diagnosis. *Hum Reprod.* 2010;25(1):275-282.

19. Munne S, Lee A, Rosenwaks Z, et al. Diagnosis of major chromosome aneuploidies in human preimplantation embryos. *Hum Reprod.* 1993;8(12):2185-2191.

20. Mastenbroek S, Twisk M, van Echten-Arends J, et al. In vitro fertilization with preimplantation genetic screening. *N Engl J Med.* 2007;357(1):9-17.

21. Schoolcraft WB, Treff NR, Stevens JM, et al. Live birth outcome with trophectoderm biopsy, blastocyst vitrification, and single-nucleotide polymorphism microarray-based comprehensive chromosome screening in infertile patients. *Fertil Steril.* 2011;96(3):638-640.

Common Fetal Malformations Diagnosed by Ultrasound

Case 1: An ultrasound performed at 20 weeks' gestation in your 21-year-old $G_2 P_1$ patient indicates an apparently isolated unilateral cleft lip/cleft palate in the fetus (Figure 10-1).

The purpose of this chapter is not to provide an in-depth discussion of particular fetal malformations, nor to cover a comprehensive list of fetal malformations. Rather our purpose is to discuss the genetic implications of common ultrasound-detected fetal malformations, and outline the general principles for evaluating and managing fetal structural abnormalities.

Cleft lip with, or without, cleft palate is one of the most common birth defects in the United States, occurring in approximately 1 in 1000 live births annually.[1] Most cases of clefting appear multifactorial; that is, a combination of genetic determinants and environmental factors. Certain medications, such as anticonvulsants, are associated with an increased risk for cleft lip/cleft palate. Likewise, poorly controlled diabetes in pregnancy can increase the risk of fetal clefts. Most importantly, a significant number of clefts, especially cleft palate, are part of a genetic syndrome, and the prognosis for the child will depend on the underlying condition, and not the severity of the cleft.

Initial evaluations should be aimed at determining if the cleft is an isolated finding.[2] Amniocentesis should be performed for standard chromosome testing and microarray testing. A fetal echocardiogram should be done to exclude cardiac malformations that would suggest a genetic syndrome. Equally important is a complete family history to determine if other family members are known to have facial clefts, or other birth defects. Counseling of the patient regarding prognosis for her child should be done by a multidisciplinary team with experience in managing infants and children with craniofacial abnormalities.

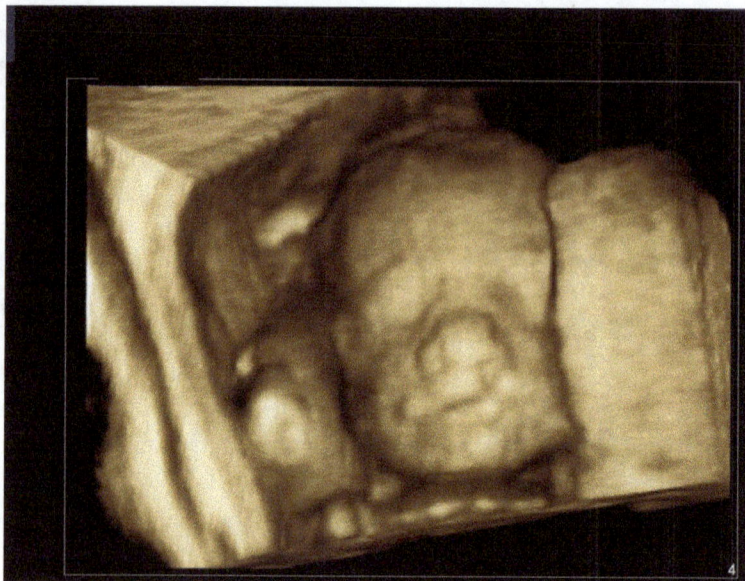

FIGURE 10-1. Three-dimensional ultrasound rendering of a fetus with a left cleft lip.

Case 2: Your 34-year-old infertility patient who conceived by ovulation induction has just had a first-trimester ultrasound indicating "fetal exencephaly." How do you counsel the patient regarding prognosis, management, and risk of recurrence in future pregnancies?

Neural tube defects (NTD) are common birth defects occurring in 1 to 2 per 1000 live births. Included in the category of NTD are anencephaly, myelomeningocele, and encephalocele. Most are characterized by multifactorial inheritance, with the one known environment factor being maternal folic acid intake. With most pregnancies now being screened by maternal serum alpha-fetoprotein (MSAFP) and/or a second trimester ultrasound, most cases of NTD are being detected *in utero*. Once the ultrasound diagnosis of a specific NTD is made, an appropriate genetic work-up should be done to provide both prognostic and recurrence risk information to the couple.

Anencephaly is characterized by a complete absence of skull development, and after the second trimester of pregnancy, absence of the cerebral hemispheres. However, on first trimester ultrasounds, fetal brain can be seen and the terms, "exencephaly" and "acrania," are often used. Both are describing what will ultimately be anencephaly. Midline defects are associated with anencephaly, including spina bifida, cleft lip/palate, and omphalocele. A small number of cases are the result of amniotic bands, and the fetus/infant should be carefully assessed for evidence of amniotic bands, as the likelihood of recurrence would be markedly less in subsequent pregnancies. Chromosome abnormalities are rarely the etiology of anencephaly, but too

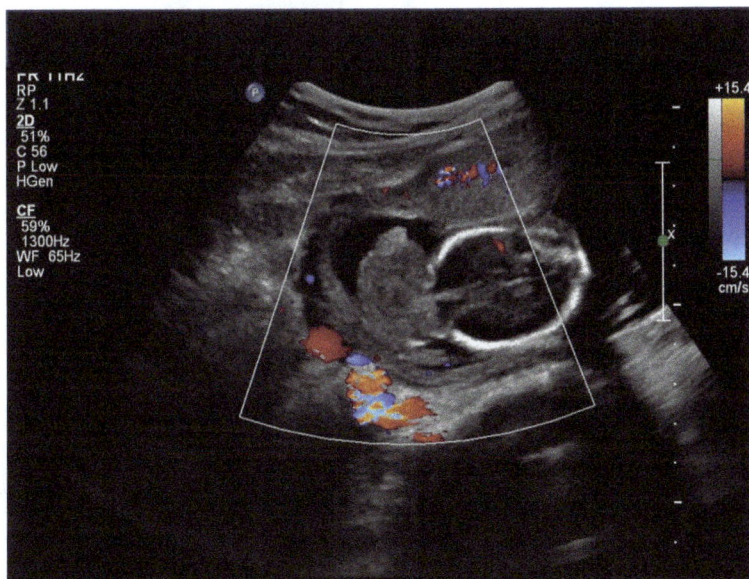

FIGURE 10-2. Ultrasound view of a large posterior fetal encephalocele.

few cases have been evaluated using microarray technology to know whether microdeletion/microduplication will be an important etiology for anencephaly.

Encephaloceles (Figure 10-2) are skull defects that allow brain tissue to protrude outside the cranial cavity. The majority are skin-covered and, therefore, will not be detected by MSAFP. Among the NTD, it is the malformation most likely to be a part of genetic syndromes, and a detailed search for other abnormalities on ultrasound, a fetal echocardiogram, and genetic studies, such as microarray testing should be performed once an encephalocele has been detected. Should the couple choose pregnancy termination, an autopsy and genetic studies likewise should be done, as recurrence risk, subsequent prenatal testing, and possible preconception therapy all depend on a precise diagnosis. For example, the genetic condition, Meckel-Gruber syndrome, is characterized by the triad of encephalocele, polycystic kidneys, and polydactyly. It is inherited in an autosomal recessive fashion with a 25% chance of recurrence, not the 2% to 3% recurrence risk for an isolated NTD. More importantly, determining the exact gene mutation would allow a precise first-trimester diagnosis by CVS, rather than depending on ultrasound in the second trimester to look for features that may have variability from one fetus to the next. In addition, recommending increased folate intake, as is appropriate in the context of a previous child with an NTD, would have no benefit in the setting of a previous pregnancy with the Meckel-Gruber syndrome.

Myelomeningocele (see Figure 10-3), or spina bifida, is the most common form of NTD. Approximately 80% of the open (non-skin covered) lesions will be detected by MSAFP, and in experienced centers ultrasound will detect more than 90%, including

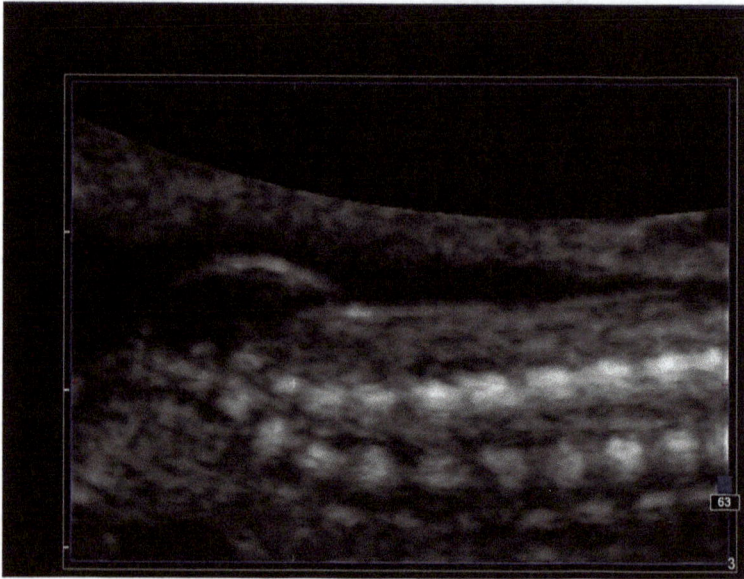

FIGURE 10-3. Second-trimester longitudinal view of a myelomeningocele sac in a low lumbo-sacral spina bifida.

many of the closed defects, because of the additional cranial findings ("lemon" sign and "banana" sign) that are associated with spina bifida. Although the majority (90%) of spina bifida cases are isolated defects, it is essential to rule out the minority that are the result of specific genetic syndrome, such as trisomy 18.[3] Chromosome studies and microarray analysis should be performed for prognosis and recurrence risk determination, and prior to any discussion of *in utero* repair options.

The counseling for this patient is that for anencephaly. It is a uniformly fatal condition, and pregnancy termination is an appropriate option. However, should she desire to continue the pregnancy, there are no significant pregnancy complications that would be associated with carrying an anencephalic fetus, other than a slightly increased risk of developing polyhydramnios, and possible preterm labor. Should she terminate, chromosome studies and microarray testing should be done. If those are negative, the risk for recurrence would be 2% to 3% for any of the NTDs. She should be given a prescription for 4 mg daily of folic acid before attempting to conceive again.

Case 3: Ms. Killian is a 28-year-old G_3P_2 whose first-trimester screen (FTS) indicated a nuchal translucency measurement of 4 mm. The FTS result indicated a risk of Down syndrome of greater than 1 in 10. After extensive counseling, Ms. Killian declined invasive testing. You have received the report from her ultrasound done at 18 weeks' gestation, which indicates an apparently isolated fetal diaphragmatic hernia. How should you counsel Ms. Killian based on this new information.

Diaphragmatic hernia (DH) is a relatively common congenital malformation occurring in approximately 1 in every 5000 live births.[1] The prognosis for the infant is dependent on the degree of pulmonary hypoplasia and on the presence, or absence, of associated abnormalities. In 30% to 40% of prenatally detected DH, there are associated malformations, with chromosomal, cardiac, central nervous system, and renal being the most common. Both trisomy 18 and 21 have been associated with DH, and a unique chromosome abnormality (isochromosome 12p), the Pallister-Killian syndrome, is seen in a significant number of prenatally diagnosed cases of DH.[4] An autosomal recessive condition, Fryns syndrome, also has DH as one of its manifestations, and like Pallister-Killian, is a lethal condition. Prior to any discussions regarding prognosis for a fetus detected with DH, there should be an amniocentesis for both routine cytogenetics, as well as microarray testing. Molecular studies for specific gene mutations may be indicated, if other abnormalities are seen on ultrasound that are suggestive of a specific syndrome. Finally, a fetal echocardiogram should be done to exclude associated cardiac abnormalities.

In counseling Ms. Killian there are several key issues. Although Down syndrome could be the underlying etiology of the fetal DH, an increased nuchal translucency can be seen in fetuses that are subsequently found to have an isolated DH. Therefore, an amniocentesis is now essential to determine the chromosome status of the fetus. Should the genetic testing be found to be negative, and no other structural malformation be found by imaging modalities, the prognosis for the infant will be determined by degree of pulmonary hypoplasia present at birth. Ms. Killian should be referred to a multidisciplinary "fetal treatment" center for further consultation and management of the pregnancy.

> **Case 4: Ms. Beckwith is a 19-year-old G₁ who presents late for prenatal care. You order a dating ultrasound that indicates a composite gestational age of 20 weeks, and a fetal abdominal wall defect with small bowel present outside the fetal abdomen (Figure 10-4). Your radiologist interprets the fetal malformation as "either a gastroschisis or ruptured omphalocele." How should you manage Ms. Beckwith's pregnancy?**

Abdominal wall defects (AWD) most commonly are either gastroschisis or omphalocele. Although the idea of a "ruptured omphalocele" is described in the pediatric surgical literature, the evidence for this occurring prenatally is exceedingly weak. Experienced radiologists are able to easily distinguish whether the AWD is a gastroschisis or omphalocele, based on classic ultrasound features, which are well described in Callen.[5] There are significant differences between the two forms of AWD both in terms of associated abnormalities, as well as the incidence of an underlying genetic etiology.

Gastroschisis is seen most commonly in young, white women in their first pregnancy, strongly suggesting both an underlying genetic predisposition, and some consistent environment factors. It is rarely associated with other structural

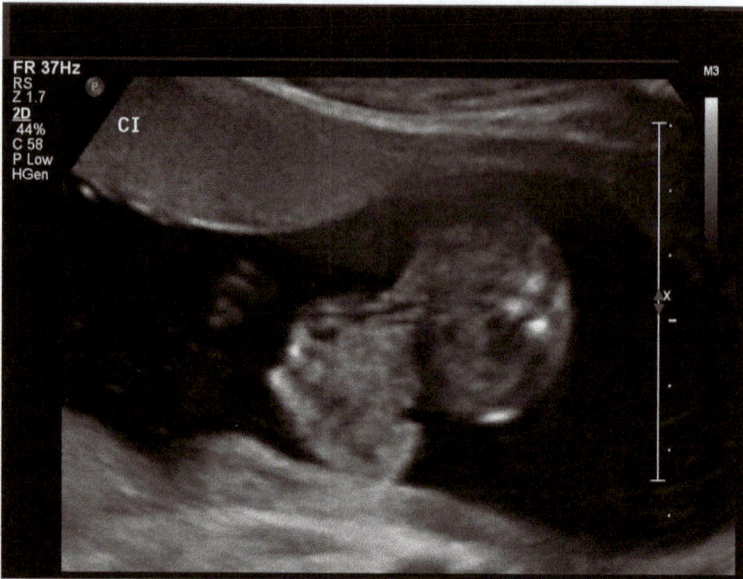

FIGURE 10-4. Ultrasound of a fetal abdominal wall defect. Absence of any covering membrane and a defect that is to the right of the umbilical cord indicate the presence of a gastroschisis.

birth defects, with intestinal malformations being the major association. There is a small increase in cardiac malformations; therefore, a fetal echocardiogram should be performed.

On the other hand, fetal omphalocele is associated with other malformations in 60% or more of prenatally detected cases. Cardiac defects and chromosomal abnormalities (trisomy 13 and 18 being the most common) make up most of the associated findings. In about 5% of cases the underlying etiology is an overgrowth syndrome, known as the Beckwith-Wiedemann syndrome, an autosomal dominant condition in some families. The manifestations of this condition are quite variable, and the only malformation in one individual may be a small umbilical hernia. Thus, it is essential to do a careful and directed family history in the evaluation of a patient whose fetus has an omphalocele. Because of the high incidence of associated abnormalities, amniocentesis should be performed for chromosome studies, microarray, and specific genetic testing for the Beckwith-Wiedemann syndrome. A fetal echocardiogram should be done to assess for cardiac malformations.

For Ms. Beckwith the key is confirming the specific AWD. Assuming the diagnosis to be a gastroschisis, no genetic testing is indicated and only a fetal echocardiogram should be done. Because of the increased risk of intrauterine growth restriction and stillbirth associated with fetal gastroschisis and the potential for significant neonatal management issues, Ms. Beckwith's pregnancy should be managed by a multidisciplinary team with experience in managing pregnancies complicated by fetal abnormalities.

> **Case 5:** Ms. Potter is a 30-year-old G_3P_2 whose family history is remarkable for a paternal grandmother who died at age 55 of kidney disease, and her father died at age 49 of a stroke. The patient is otherwise healthy and her two previous pregnancies were uncomplicated, and resulted in full-term vaginal deliveries of healthy infants. You have just received her ultrasound report that was performed at 20 weeks' gestation based on a known last menstrual period. The report indicates fetal biometry consistent with her menstrual dating. There is no measurable amniotic fluid, and both fetal kidneys are described as large containing multiple large cysts. The radiologist's impression is "infantile with disease." Do you agree with the diagnosis? What are the next steps in the diagnostic evaluation?

Cystic kidneys is a generic term used in fetal sonography that can include disorders ranging from severe hydronephrosis to multicystic dysplastic kidneys (MCDK). The term gives neither prognostic information, nor information on the underlying etiology. The first step in the evaluation of apparently cystic kidneys is to look for evidence of obstruction at the three sites where blockage can occur (urethra, ureteropelvic junction, and ureterovesical junction). Once obstruction has been identified, standard management protocols should be followed (see Bianchi or Sanders).[1,3] Chromosome abnormalities are a relatively common etiology for urethral obstruction, but are rare in fetuses with either ureterovesical or ureteropelvic junction obstruction.

Once obstruction has been excluded, then the remaining issue is to determine whether the "cysts" are part of an isolated renal disease, or are part of a genetic syndrome. Large cysts in the fetal kidneys are usually the result of the disorder known as **multicystic dysplastic kidneys**, which can be either unilateral or bilateral. It is a sporadic disorder, thought to be a result of failure to develop a normal connection between the anlage of the fetal kidney and the fetal ureter (a small atretic ureter is often found with the enlarged cystic kidney). MCDK are most commonly characterized by multiple cysts of varying sizes, interspersed in solid material that represents the dysplastic component of the kidney (Figure 10-5). The overall shape of the kidney can vary significantly, and the kidney may be quite large, and in the case of bilateral disease, the two MCDK may fill the abdomen. Because the MCDK are nonfunctional, bilateral disease is associated with absence of amniotic fluid, and neonatal death from pulmonary hypoplasia. On the other hand, unilateral MCDK has an excellent prognosis, assuming no other pathology is found in the contralateral kidney.[6]

Adult polycystic kidney disease (APKD) is an autosomal dominant condition, characterized by single, or multiple cysts, in kidneys of normal size and shape. Most individuals who inherit the gene will develop renal cysts in their late 20s, and will generally progress to end-stage renal disease over the next few decades. There

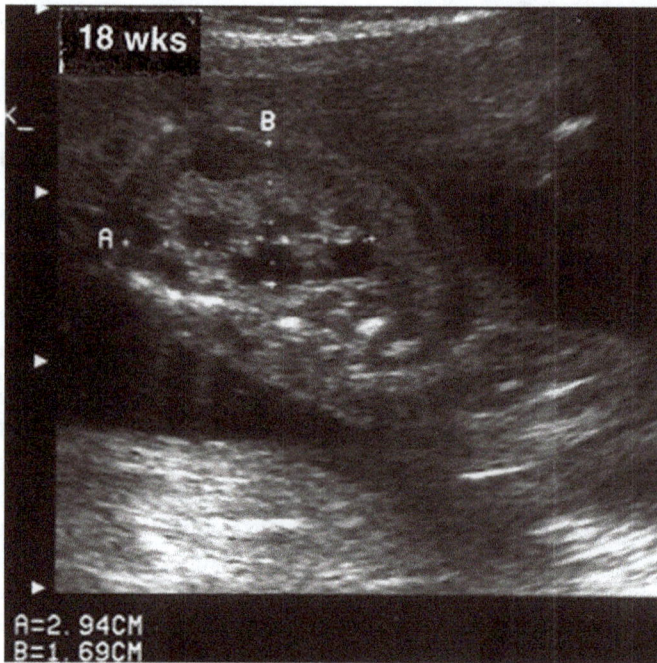

FIGURE 10-5. Ultrasound of typical multicystic dysplastic kidney with cysts of varying sizes interspersed in dysplastic appearing renal parenchyma.

is an association of the disease also with cerebral aneurysms and stroke resulting from rupture of the aneurysm. In approximately 10% of individuals who inherit the APKD genes (PKD1, PKD2), the disease will present in the fetal or neonatal period with cystic kidneys, renal failure, and, if early in the fetal period, anhydramnios and resultant pulmonary hypoplasia, and neonatal death. Depending on the age of the parents, there may, or may not, be cysts in the kidneys of the parent who has transmitted the gene. Generally, the kidneys in a fetus with APKD will be more reniform in appearance, but in more severe cases may be indistinguishable from the appearance of bilateral MCDK. In the absence of amniotic fluid, the prognosis will be the same in both conditions. For subsequent pregnancies, it is essential that a precise diagnosis be established.

Infantile polycystic kidney disease (IPKD) is an autosomal recessive disease. The kidneys in IPKD are characterized by multiple small cysts that are below the resolution of ultrasound (Figure 10-6). Therefore, a fetal kidney affected by IPKD will appear quite large and echogenic. It is a bilateral disease process, and the presence of these two large structures often will fill the fetal abdomen, and result in a significant increase in abdominal circumference. Because the kidneys have some function, amniotic fluid volume often will be normal. It should be noted that the kidneys in trisomy 13 and the Meckel-Gruber syndrome can have an identical

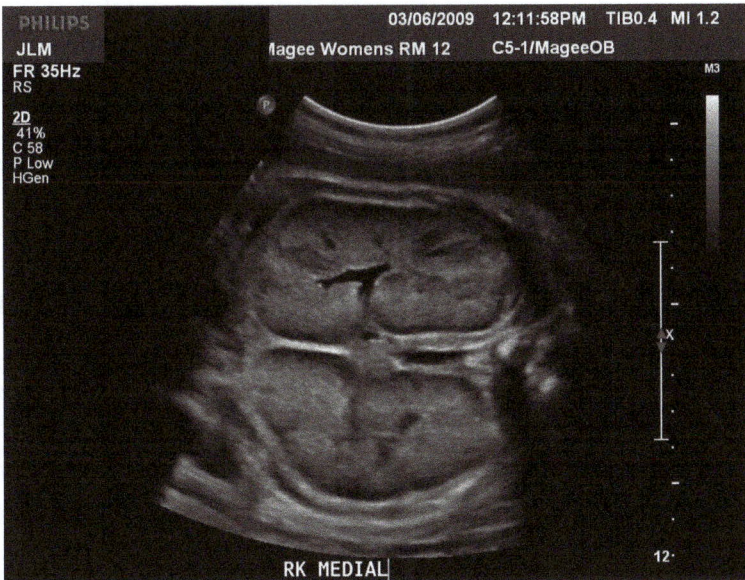

FIGURE 10-6. Ultrasound of bilateral infantile polycystic kidneys in a second trimester fetus. Note the increased echogenicity, large size, and relatively normal reniform appearance.

appearance to IPKD. Therefore, a precise diagnosis must be made before it is possible to discuss prognosis and management, and is key to determining risk for recurrence in subsequent pregnancies.

In counseling Ms. Potter, the family history gives strong clues for a possible diagnosis of APKD (kidney failure, strokes). Although MCDK disease cannot be excluded, it is possible to exclude the diagnosis of IPKD based on the "multiple large cysts" seen on ultrasound. The first step in further evaluation is to assess Ms. Potter's kidneys, as more than 90% of those with the gene mutation will have renal cysts by age 30.[3] The absence of cysts in Ms. Potter's kidneys does not exclude the diagnosis of APKD, and genetic testing should be done on her to look for the gene mutation. If she has an APKD mutation, subsequent pregnancies can be tested in the first trimester with CVS, or Ms. Potter could choose preimplantation genetic diagnosis. In addition, Ms. Potter should be referred to a nephrologist for continued management of APKD.

This chapter has not attempted to be all-inclusive in its discussion of fetal malformations, but rather has as its objective to remind the reader of the strong association between structural abnormalities in the fetus, and genetic conditions. As a rule of thumb, when a malformation is detected on ultrasound evaluation, it should be assumed not to be isolated until a thorough genetic evaluation has been done. Even then, the patient should be cautioned that many genetic disorders will not have obvious fetal structural malformations, and that any genetic testing is limited by the differential diagnosis that prompted a specific genetic test. Even a comprehensive evaluation at birth may not detect the presence of a condition that will have its full manifestation later in childhood.

REFERENCES

1. Sanders RC, Blackmon LR, Hogge WA, Wulfsberg EA. *Structural Fetal Abnormalities: The Total Picture.* St. Louis, MO: Mosby; 2002.

2. Benacerraf BB. The Sherlock Holmes approach to diagnosing fetal syndromes by ultrasound. *Clin Obstet Gynecol.* 2012;55:226-248.

3. Bianchi DW, Crombleholme TM, D'Alton ME, Malone FD. *Fetology: Diagnosis and Management of the Fetal Patient.* 2nd ed. New York, NY: McGraw-Hill; 2010.

4. Benacerraf B. *Ultrasound of Fetal Syndromes.* 2nd ed. Philadelphia, PA: Churchill Livingstone Elsevier; 2008.

5. Callen PW. *Ultrasonography in Obstetrics and Gynecology.* 5th ed. Philadelphia, PA: Saunders Elsevier; 2008.

6. Naimi AAI, Baumuller, JE, Spahn S, Bahlmann F. Prenatal diagnosis of multicystic dysplastic kidney disease in the second trimester screening. *Prenat Diagn.* 2013;32:1-6.

Gynecologic Disorders With a Genetic Causation

- LEIOMYOMAS
- MENARCHE AND MENOPAUSE
- POLYCYSTIC OVARIAN SYNDROME
- ENDOMETRIOSIS
- CLINICAL CONSIDERATIONS

Case 1: Ms. Kolthoff is a 27-year-old $G_0 P_0$, who was evaluated for accelerated growth and advanced bone age in high school. She is currently married without children. She does not use birth control and despite sexual intercourse approximately a few times a week for the past 2 years, she has not conceived. She complains of having to shave her upper lip as well as hair on her back and abdomen. Her menstrual cycles are irregular and she sometimes will not have one for several months. She has experienced acne for which she took over-the-counter lotions for treatment with partial success, and was also given a short course of antibiotics by her physician. She has been told she has polycystic ovarian syndrome, and presents with concerns about her fertility. Her family history is unremarkable. She has three sisters who do not have hirsutism, and all three have children. The physical exam was significant for short stature, shaved upper lip, acne-related facial scarring, and significant abdominal and back hirsutism. Her external genitalia appeared normal and the pelvic exam was unremarkable. A basal 17-hydroxyprogesterone measure was 1850 ng/dL, while an ACTH stimulation test showed a 17-hydroxyprogesterone rise to 5300 ng/dL. What additional tests and evaluation would you consider for Ms. Kolthoff?

Gynecologic disorders can be heritable, such as polycystic ovarian syndrome, or can be due to sporadic somatic mutations that arise in individual organs, such as uterine leiomyomas. To date gene mutations have been associated with common gynecologic disorders, such as leiomyomas, polycystic ovarian syndrome, endometriosis, and menstrual dysfunction. We also know that specific genomic regions regulate important reproductive landmarks, such as menarche and menopause. In the future, genomic medicine will play a significant role in understanding the causation of gynecologic disorders and guiding individual therapies.

■ LEIOMYOMAS

Leiomyomas, or fibroids, are common tumors arising from the myometrial layer of the uterus. They are clinically diagnosed in 25% of women, and are often associated with dysmenorrhea, menorrhagia, infertility, and abdominal discomfort. Subclinical leiomyomas are extremely common, and by age 50 more than 80% of black and 70% of white women have leiomyomas. Family history, black race, age, nulliparity, and obesity are known risk factors for the development of clinically significant leiomyomas. Family aggregation and twin studies show that genes contribute significantly to the genesis of leiomyomas.[1] Common leiomyomas are monoclonal in origin, and 40% have associated chromosome abnormalities. Cytogenetic aberrations commonly include deletions in 7q, trisomy of chromosome 12, and various translocations between chromosomes 12 and 14 involving the high-mobility group AT-hook 2 (HMGA2) gene at 12q15, which encodes a transcriptional regulator. Cytogenetic abnormalities are likely a reflection of general genomic instability, as is true for other tumors. Individuals may have leiomyomas either due to germline mutations (rare) or due to somatic mutations that arise only in the uterus (common).

Heterozygous (present on one allele) germline mutations in fumarate hydratase (FH) predispose individuals to a rare disorder known as hereditary cutaneous and uterine leiomyomatosis with renal carcinoma (OMIM 150800).[2] This disorder follows the classic Knudson "two-hit" model, where affected individuals carry a mutation in one allele in all tissues, and a second mutation is acquired in affected tissues to cause leiomyomatosis and renal cancer. Fumarate hydratase acts, therefore, as a tumor suppressor gene. However, fumarate hydratase mutations are not the cause of common leiomyomas.

Genomewide association studies have identified several genomic locations that associate with leiomyomas. Three loci on chromosomes 10q24.33, 22q13.1, and 11p15.5 were associated with clinically significant uterine fibroids in Japanese women,[3] and seven loci on chromosomes 10p11, 3p21, 2q37, 5p13, 11p15, 12q14, and 17q25 were associated with leiomyomas in Caucasian women.[4] The fatty acid synthase gene (FASN) is located on 17q25 and overexpressed in leiomyomas as compared to normal myometrium. FASN has been implicated in progression of other tumors, and possibly may provide a biologic link to leiomyomatous growth, although mechanistic evidence for it is lacking. Overall, it remains unclear how these loci influence leiomyomatous growth.

Somatic mutations in the MED12 gene (mediator complex subunit 12; located on Xq13.1) are associated with common leiomyomas.[5,6] These mutations are present only in leiomyomas, but not in the surrounding, normal myometrial tissues. MED12 mutations cluster in exon 2, and the mechanisms by which these mutations arise in the myometrium are not well understood. Overall, MED12 was mutated in 100/148 (67%) of the genotyped leiomyomas: 79/148 (53%) leiomyomas exhibited heterozygous missense single nucleotide variants, 17/148 (11%) leiomyomas exhibited heterozygous in-frame deletions/insertion-deletions, 2/148 (1%) leiomyomas exhibited intronic heterozygous single nucleotide variants affecting splicing, and 2/148 (1%) leiomyomas exhibited heterozygous deletions/insertion-deletions spanning the intron 1 to exon 2 boundary which affected the splice acceptor site. The most commonly observed nonsynonymous SNP was the c.131G>A heterozygous mutation causing a glycine to aspartic acid amino acid change. MED12 mutations were equally distributed among karyotypically normal and abnormal uterine leiomyomas and were identified in leiomyomas from both black and white American women. It is, therefore, likely that MED12 variants deregulate the cell cycle in the normal myometrium, resulting in abnormal growth, genomic instability, and karyotype abnormalities in a subset of leiomyomas. The karyotype abnormalities are, therefore, a consequence of MED12 mutations, rather than cause of uterine leiomyomas. MED12 is a 250 kilodalton (kDa) protein, which is part of a large complex of mediator proteins, and is involved in transcriptional regulation of RNA polymerase II complex. This complex is highly conserved among all eukaryotes, and is involved in both repression and activation of DNA transcription as well as chromatin remodeling. MED12 is located on the X chromosome, and naturally occurring random X chromosome inactivation allows gene expression from only one of the X chromosomes. The X chromosome that carries the MED12 mutation is expressed in leiomyomas, meaning that altered MED12 protein is produced and causes tumorigenesis. Not all leiomyomas carry MED12 mutations, and therefore other mechanisms exist that lead to leiomyoma formation.

■ MENARCHE AND MENOPAUSE

Menarche and menopause are important landmarks in a woman's reproductive life, and overall health. Their onset is dependent on the interplay of both environmental and genetic factors. Heritability estimates from twin and family studies are 50% for age at natural menopause and menarche, and indicate the great importance of genes in these two events. The timing of menarche and menopause has important implications for a number of diseases. Early onset of menarche and late onset of menopause are associated with increased risks of breast, ovarian and endometrial cancer. Later onset of menarche is associated with a decreased risk of obesity, and diabetes, and decreased fertility. Early onset of menopause is associated with decreased fertility, an increased risk of osteoporosis, and an increased risk of cardiovascular disease.

Genomewide association studies have shown that genetic markers in the vicinity of the height-related gene, LIN28B, as well as 31 other loci, are associated with menarche.[7] The genes that associate with menarche are important in the regulation of body mass index (FTO, SEC16B, TRA2B, and TMEM18), energy homeostasis (BSX, CRTC1, and MCHR2), hormonal regulation (INHBA, PCSK2, and RXRG), and fatty acid biosynthesis. Having 32 different loci associated with the age of menarche indicates that multiple pathways are involved in the initiation of menarche.

Genomewide association studies have implicated 18 different loci in the age of onset of menopause.[8,9] These loci include genes implicated in DNA repair (MCM8, MSH6, EXO1, HELQ, UIMC1, FAM175A, FANCI, TLK1, and PRIM1), and immune (IL11, NLRP11, and PRRC2A) and mitochondrial function (POLG). Early menopause, defined as menopause that occurs at less than 45 years of age, is also associated with genetic loci that govern the onset of menopause. DNA repair genes are involved in many of the disorders of early aging, and it is likely that a subset of women with early menopause, or premature ovarian insufficiency, are at risk for accelerated aging and early death. For example, women with Fanconi anemia have mutations in DNA repair genes and suffer from accelerated aging, early menopause, hormonal dysfunction, and a propensity to develop tumors. Women who show signs of accelerated aging and premature ovarian insufficiency should be evaluated to rule out heritable genetic syndromes. Despite the impressive number of loci associated with the onset of menarche and menopause, these loci probably account for less than 15% of the estimated genetic contribution. These results are not unexpected, because we know from animal models that many more genes are involved in determining the reproductive life span.

■ POLYCYSTIC OVARIAN SYNDROME

Polycystic ovarian syndrome (PCOS) is a relatively common gynecologic disorder that affects as many as 8% of women of childbearing age, and is characterized by hyperandrogenism, ovulatory dysfunction, and polycystic ovaries. Women with PCOS commonly present with menstrual disorders, and are subfertile. Hirsutism and acne are common skin manifestations, and likely due to peripheral androgen excess. PCOS also increases the risk for endometrial cancer, type 2 diabetes, hypertension, hyperlipidemia, and cardiovascular disorders.[10] The PCOS phenotype can be caused by various genetic defects. One example is nonclassical congenital adrenal hyperplasia, a heritable,[11] autosomal recessive disorder. It is relatively common among Ashkenazi Jews, Hispanics, Native American Inuits in Alaska, and Italians (incidence of approximately 3%). Although caused by mutations in the 21-hydroxylase gene, unlike classic adrenal hyperplasia, the mutations have milder effects on the enzyme action, and cause a less severe phenotype, manifesting as PCOS. Nonclassical congenital adrenal hyperplasia is best diagnosed by measuring serum 17-hydroxyprogesterone levels which are elevated following stimulation with adrenocorticotropic hormone (ACTH). Women who are diagnosed with nonclassical congenital adrenal hyperplasia should have the 21 hydroxylase gene sequenced to determine their mutation status. If positive for a known mutation, their partner should also be tested to determine if they are at risk to have a child with the classical form of congenital adrenal hyperplasia.

Most of the PCOS cases are idiopathic, and do not appear to follow simple Mendelian inheritance. PCOS is, like many gynecologic disorders, a complex condition, and genomewide association studies have identified 11 loci that associate with PCOS.[12] Genes in these loci are involved in insulin signaling pathways (INSR), ovulatory function (FSHR, LHCGR), and type 2 diabetes (THADA). The identification of these genes and their related pathways will allow better understanding of PCOS, and result in more rational therapies in the future.

ENDOMETRIOSIS

Endometriosis is a common gynecologic disorder that affects approximately 5% to 10% of reproductive age women. Endometriosis is characterized by implantation of endometrial tissue outside of the uterus. Women with endometriosis may complain of dysmenorrhea (painful menstruation), dyspareunia (pain during sexual intercourse), dysuria (pain during urination), dyschezia (difficulty with defecating) and infertility. Family-based studies have shown that first-degree relatives of women with endometriosis are approximately 6 times more likely to have endometriosis then women with a negative family history.[13] It also appears that familial endometriosis presents with more significant symptoms. Twin studies have shown a high concordance (50%) of endometriosis in monozygotic (genetically identical twins), as opposed to dizygotic twins.[14] The family based and monozygotic twin pairs studies are consistent with the interpretation that an individual's genome contributes significantly to the risk of developing endometriosis.

Identification of genes responsible for endometriosis has not been easy, due to the complexity of the disease, and the likely contribution of multiple genes. Genomewide association studies on Japanese and Caucasian women have identified at least seven genomic loci on chromosomes 7p15.2, 1p36.12, 2p25.1, 12q22, 2p14, 6p22.3, and 9p21.3. Numerous genes are located in these loci, some of which are biologically connected to the reproductive tract. These include WNT4, GREB1, and VEZT. WNT4 is important for the development of the female reproductive tract and for steroidogenesis. Another interesting gene is GREB1 which encodes a protein that is involved in hormone-dependent breast cancer cell growth. VEZT encodes an adherens junction transmembrane protein, and may play a role as a tumor suppressor gene.[15] Much work remains to be done to determine what role these genes may play in the development of endometriosis.

CLINICAL CONSIDERATIONS

Women that present with gynecologic disorders should have a three-generation pedigree obtained that elicits the medical problems, including the gynecologic disorder under investigation, for all family members. For the particular gynecologic disorder, it is important to note the age of onset, severity, treatment, and response to therapy. A family history in women with gynecologic disorders is important to determine whether the condition is familial, and the apparent mode of inheritance. Genetic testing should be reserved for conditions that can have important implications for the family unit, offspring, and/or disease management decisions. There are very few clinical genetic tests geared toward gynecologic disorders, as our current knowledge about reproductive genetics does not allow for differential management based on an individual's genotype. The recent identification of many genetic loci that associate with various gynecologic conditions, as well as future application of this knowledge to medical management, may allow for more individualized medical therapies.

In the vignette at the beginning of this chapter, the 17-hydroxyprogesterone levels with, and without, ACTH stimulation are consistent with a diagnosis of the nonclassical form of congenital adrenal hyperplasia. These individuals are at risk to have a child with classic form of congenital adrenal hyperplasia, and should undergo genetic testing for mutations in the 21-hydroxylase gene. Genetic testing revealed that Ms. Kolthoff carried a classic mutation on one allele, and mild mutation on another allele. She understood that her future partner should be tested to determine whether he is a carrier for a classic congenital adrenal hyperplasia mutation. Her anovulation was successfully treated within 3 months of initiating dexamethasone therapy.

REFERENCES

1. Ligon AH, Morton CC. Leiomyomata: heritability and cytogenetic studies. *Hum. Reprod Update.* 2001;7:8-14.
2. Tomlinson IP, Alam NA, Rowan AJ, et al. Germline mutations in FH predispose to dominantly inherited uterine fibroids, skin leiomyomata and papillary renal cell cancer. *Nat Genet.* 2002;4:406-410.
3. Cha PC, Takahashi A, Hosono N, et al. A genomewide association study identifies three loci associated with susceptibility to uterine fibroids. *Nat Genet.* 2011;43: 447-450.
4. Eggert SL, Huyck KL, Somasundaram P, et al. Genomewide linkage and association analyses implicate FASN in predisposition to Uterine Leiomyomata. *Am J Hum Genet.* 2012;91:621-628.
5. Makinen N, Mehine M, Tolvanen J, et al. MED12, the mediator complex subunit 12 gene, is mutated at high frequency in uterine leiomyomas. *Science.* 2011;334:252-255.
6. McGuire MM, Yatsenko A, Hoffner L, Jones M, Surti U, Rajkovic A. Whole exome sequencing in a random sample of North American women with leiomyomas identifies MED12 mutations in majority of uterine leiomyomas. *PloS One.* 2012;7:e33251.
7. Elks CE, Perry JR, Sulem P, et al. Thirty new loci for age at menarche identified by a meta-analysis of genomewide association studies. *Nat Genet.* 2010;42:1077-1085.
8. Stolk L, Perry JR, Chasman DI, et al. Meta-analyses identify 13 loci associated with age at menopause and highlight DNA repair and immune pathways. *Nat Genet.* 2012;44:260-268.
9. Perry JR, Hsu YH, Chasman DI, et al. DNA mismatch repair gene MSH6 implicated in determining age at natural menopause. *Hum Mol Genet.* 2014, Jan 8.

10. ACOG Practice Bulletin No. 108. Polycystic ovary syndrome. *Obstet Gynecol.* 2009;114:936-949.

11. New MI. Extensive clinical experience: nonclassical 21-hydroxylase deficiency. *J Clin Endocrinol Metab.* 2006;91:4205-4214.

12. Shi Y, Han Z, Yuhua S, et al. Genomewide association study identifies eight new risk loci for polycystic ovary syndrome. *Nat Genet.* 2012;44:1020-1025.

13. Simpson JL, Elias S, Malinak LR, Buttram VC Jr. Heritable aspects of endometriosis. I. Genetic studies. *Am J Obstet Gynecol.* 1980;137:327-331.

14. Treloar SA, O'Connor DT, O'Connor VM, Martin NG. Genetic influences on endometriosis in an Australian twin sample. *Fertil Steril.* 1999;71:701-710.

15. Miao R, Guo X, Zhi Q, et al. VEZT, a novel putative tumor suppressor, suppresses the growth and tumorigenicity of gastric cancer. *PloS One.* 2013;8:e74409.

Hereditary Cancer Syndromes

■ **HEREDITARY CANCER SYNDROMES**

Hereditary Breast and Ovarian Cancer

Hereditary Nonpolyposis Colon Cancer (Lynch Syndrome)

Li-Fraumeni Syndrome

Cowden Syndrome

Hereditary Leiomyomatosis and Renal Cell Cancer

General Considerations

Overview of Genetic Testing

> **Case 1: A 25-year-old patient presents to you for an annual examination. Evaluation of her family history reveals that her paternal grandmother and a paternal aunt died of breast cancer in their early 40s.**

Screening for familial cancer is an important part of the initial evaluation of a patient, and should be a regular part of each subsequent visit to assess any changes in the family history. Obstetricians and gynecologists have an important role in identifying those women with a potentially hereditary cancer syndrome. Although it is not expected that the practicing OB/GYN would be familiar with all the hereditary cancer syndromes, they should be able to recognize the key features in a family history that suggest the patient may be at risk, and make an appropriate referral for evaluation and counseling. This chapter will outline some common hereditary cancer syndromes likely to be seen by the OB/GYN, and provide a list of key features present in families with hereditary forms of cancer.

■ HEREDITARY CANCER SYNDROMES

Hereditary Breast and Ovarian Cancer

This is a dominantly inherited syndrome most commonly caused by germline mutations in the genes *BRCA1* and *2*. In the general population the mutated gene is found in approximately 1 in every 500 persons, but in those of Ashkenazi Jewish ancestry the cancer frequency is 1 in every 40 individuals.[1] However, the majority of breast and ovarian cancers are sporadic, with only 5% to 10% of them being caused by a *BRCA1* or *2* mutation.

Key features strongly suggestive of a *BRCA1* or *2* mutation would be early onset of breast or ovarian cancer in a patient (prior to age 50), a family history with multiple affected members, or the presence in the family history of both breast and ovarian cancer. It is important to recognize that males who carry one of these mutations may be asymptomatic, but also are at risk for breast, prostate, and pancreatic cancer. Even in women with the mutation, the gene is not completely penetrant. For a female with the mutation there is 40% to 66% lifetime risk of breast cancer, and up to a 46% risk of ovarian cancer. These risks are significantly higher than the US general population risk of 12% for breast cancer and 1.5% for ovarian cancer. In addition, many of these cancers will occur before the age of 50.[2] Equally of concern is the risk of breast cancer in the contralateral breast which is between 40% and 65% over a lifetime, and up to 30% 10 years postdiagnosis.[3]

Patients with early onset breast or ovarian cancer, or those with family histories similar to that seen in the case study, should be referred to individuals trained in cancer genetic counseling for evaluation and genetic testing. If the patient is found to carry a pathogenic mutation, an appropriate management plan needs to be developed to include both screening options and prophylactic surgical options (mastectomy and oophorectomy).

The absence of a known pathogenic mutation does not exclude the possibility that the family has a hereditary form of breast and/or ovarian cancer. In addition to the other known syndromes outlined below, there are likely many other cancer causing gene mutations that have yet to be discovered. In the presence of a strong family history, but negative gene testing, it is essential that a comprehensive screening plan be developed for the potentially at-risk patient.

Hereditary Nonpolyposis Colon Cancer (Lynch Syndrome)

Although colon cancer is the third leading cause of cancer death in women, the great majority will be late-onset cancers. A family history of early onset colon cancer, and other cancers, such as ovarian or endometrial, should raise suspicion of Lynch syndrome, and prompt a referral for genetic counseling and gene testing for the DNA mismatch genes that are commonly mutated in this disorder. In addition to the associated gynecologic cancers, a wide variety of other cancers may be found in these families, including gastric, small intestine, biliary, brain, skin, and pancreas. In the patient identified with the Lynch syndrome a comprehensive screening plan including both a gastroenterologist and a gynecologist is essential, as the risk for ovarian cancer and endometrial cancer may be up to 12% and 60%, respectively.[4]

Li-Fraumeni Syndrome

This condition is highly penetrant with a 90% risk of cancer by age 60. Most cases are due to germline mutations in the tumor suppression genes, *p53* and *CHEK2*. Soft tissue sarcomas, often expressed in children or young adults, are the most common cancers. However, breast cancer is a commonly associated cancer, as are bone, brain, and adrenal cancers. Unlike most of the other cancer-predisposition genes the frequency of *de novo* mutations is quite high (7%-20%). In certain circumstances, gene testing may be offered in the absence of a positive family history.[5]

Cowden Syndrome

Although a relatively rare condition (1 in every 200,000 persons), this syndrome should be suspected when there is strong family history of both breast and thyroid cancer. Its unique features, which include macrocephaly and facial and mucous membrane papules, are almost always present by age 30. In addition to the 25% to 50% risk of breast cancer, there is a 5% to 10% risk of endometrial cancer. Approximately 80% of patients with Cowden syndrome are found to have a mutation in the *PTEN* gene.[6] Family history may not play as important a role in Cowden syndrome, as 50% of patients do not have a history of other affected family members.

Hereditary Leiomyomatosis and Renal Cell Cancer

This disorder is extremely rare among women with fibroids, but essentially all women with hereditary leiomyomatosis and renal cell cancer (HLRCC) have fibroids, and 75% have cutaneous leiomyomas. The fibroids tend to be present early in life, even prior to age 20, and tend to be large, numerous, and symptomatic. Approximately 10% to 15% of women with the HLRCC mutation will have renal tumors, most commonly papillary renal cell carcinoma. The gene mutation is in the *FH* gene which codes for the enzyme, fumarate hydratase.

General Considerations

Patient with family history or a personal history of early onset cancers, bilateral cancers in paired organs, male breast cancer, or cancer affecting multiple generations should be referred for genetic counseling. Table 12-1 outlines current indications to refer a patient for cancer genetic counseling. Current guidelines suggest that even in the absence of any family history of breast or ovarian cancer that patients with ovarian, primary peritoneal, and fallopian tube cancers should be referred for genetic counseling and possible *BRCA1* and *2* mutation testing. In patients of Ashkenazi Jewish descent a personal history of breast cancer at any age may be considered an indication for genetic testing.[7] Assessing both the maternal and paternal family history is important because the gene mutation, although inherited in an autosomal dominant fashion, may not manifest in a male. Genetic counseling provides the patient a detailed risk assessment, options for genetic

■ **TABLE 12-1.** Indications to Refer Patients for Genetic Counseling

- Breast cancer at ≤ 45 years of age
- Two primary breast cancers
- Male breast cancer
- Breast cancer at ≤ 50 years of age with one or more close (1st or 2nd degree) relatives with breast cancer
- Breast cancer at ≤ age 50 years with one or more close relatives with ovarian cancer
- Breast cancer with one or more of the following cancers on the same side of the family: sarcoma, brain tumor, thyroid cancer, leukemia, lymphoma, endometrial cancer, pancreatic cancer, gastric cancer
- Ovarian cancer at any age
- Colon or endometrial cancer at <50 years of age, or both cancers at any age
- Personal history of multiple primary cancers

testing, and appropriate interpretation of the results of testing, if done. Patients found to be at risk for a hereditary cancer syndrome should be managed by a multidisciplinary team with expertise in cancer genetics.

Overview of Genetic Testing

When a decision is made to proceed with genetic testing, the testing should first be offered to the person affected by the cancer in question. If that person is positive for one of the known gene mutations, then precise testing is available for other potentially at-risk, but unaffected, individuals. Equally important for the person affected is the information that a positive test puts them at risk for a second primary cancer, and that an appropriate surveillance plan must be put in place.

If a mutation is identified in the family, a negative test in other relatives removes them from the high-risk category. On the other hand, they remain at risk for sporadic cancers, and should have screening that is appropriate for the general population. A positive test for a *BRCA1* or *BRCA2* mutation requires a multidisciplinary approach to management. Table 12-2 outlines a sample management plan, but these guidelines can change rapidly and consultation with a cancer genetics professional should always precede implementing any management plan. In addition to the development of a management plan, cancer geneticists can address any psychological effects of a positive diagnosis, and provide information to the patient on the implications for other family members who may be at risk. The physician should emphasize the need to share the genetic information with all family members who may be at risk.

There are two problematic areas in genetic testing. The first is that of the "indeterminate negative." In these families, the family history is strongly suggestive of autosomal dominant inheritance, but no causative mutation is found in the family. These patients should be cautioned against interpreting the failure to find a mutation as a negative result. These patients should be treated as

■ **TABLE 12-2.** Management of a Patient with *BRCA1* and *BRCA2* Mutation*

Breast Cancer Screening

- Breast self-exam (monthly), beginning at age 18
- Frequent clinician performed breast exams, beginning at age 25
- Mammography (every 6-12 months), beginning at age 25 and consideration of breast magnetic resonance imaging

Ovarian Cancer Screening

- Pelvic exam, every 6-12 months, beginning by age 25
- CA-125 blood tests, every 6-12 months, by age 35
- Transvaginal ultrasound with color Doppler, every 6-12 months, by age 35

Breast Cancer Risk Reduction

- Consideration of chemoprevention after age 35 (eg, tamoxifen)
- Oophorectomy, if premenopausal (see below)
- Consideration of prophylactic mastectomy

Ovarian Cancer Risk Reduction

- Consideration of chemoprevention with oral contraceptives
- Prophylactic oophorectomy by age 40 or after childbearing is completed is strongly recommended

---

*Modified from Peshkin and Isaacs.[2]

high-risk patients with increased surveillance, despite the absence of a common genetic mutation.

The second area of confusion for patients is the "indeterminate positive" result. Full sequencing of *BRCA1* or *BRCA2*, as well as other cancer susceptibility genes, may detect variants of uncertain clinical significance (VUS). These variants, often a single nucleotide change, have an unknown impact on protein function. Population studies will, in some cases, identify the variant as either benign or deleterious, but most will not have been categorized. In general the finding of a VUS should not be used to modify the care of a patient or her family.

In this case scenario, the patient was referred to the local Cancer Genetics Program, and a three-generation pedigree (Figure 12-1) was obtained. In addition to the two relatives with breast cancer, she gave a history that her 40-year-old cousin had recently been diagnosed with stage III ovarian cancer. Testing of the cousin had been done as part of her evaluation, and she had been found to carry a *BRCA1* mutation. After an extensive counseling session regarding the limitations and benefits of molecular testing, our patient had *BRCA1* testing for the family-specific mutation. She did not have the mutation, but was counseled regarding the population risk for breast and ovarian cancer, and told about current screening guidelines for these cancers.

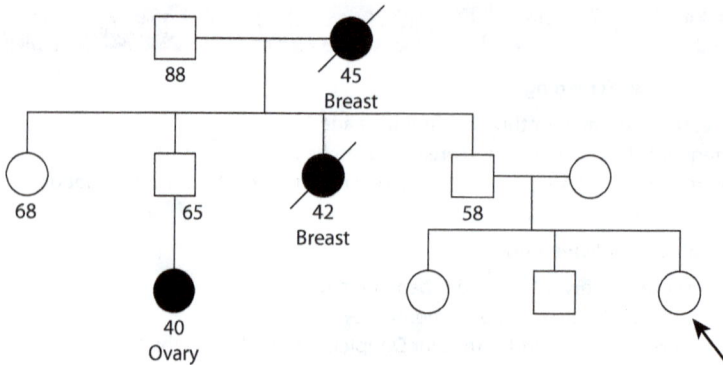

FIGURE 12-1. Three-generation pedigree of a family with strong family history of breast and ovarian cancer. Clear symbol = unaffected; filled symbol = affected with cancer; age = either current age or age at diagnosis of cancer.

REFERENCES

1. Kurian AW. *BRCA1* and *BRCA2* mutations across race and ethnicity: distribution and clinical implications. *Cur Opin Obstet Gynecol.* 2010;22(1):72-78.

2. Peshkin BN, Isaacs C. Evaluation and management of women with BRCA1/2 mutations. *Oncology.* 2005;19:1451-1459.

3. Chen S, Parmigiani G. Meta-analysis of *BRCA1* and *BRCA2* penetrance. *J Clin Oncol.* 2007;25(11):1329-1333.

4. Aarnio M, Sankila R, Pukkala E, et al. Cancer risk in mutation carriers of DNA-mismatch-repair genes. *Int J Cancer.* 1999;81(2):214-218.

5. Gonzalez KD, Buzin CH, Noltner KA, et al. High frequency of de novo mutations in Li-Fraumeni syndrome. *J Med Genet.* 2009;46(10):689-693.

6. Pilarski R, Eng C. Will the real Cowden syndrome please stand up (again)? Expanding mutational and clinical spectra of the PTEN hamartoma tumour syndrome. *J Med Genet.* 2004;41(5):323-326.

7. Daly MB, Axilbund JE, Buys S, et al. Genetic/familial high-risk assessment: breast and ovarian. *J Natl Compr Canc Netw.* 2010;8(5):562-594.

Disorders of Sexual Differentiation

Case 1: Ms. Omotoya Bamidele is a 28-year-old medical student of Yoruban origin who presented to her OB/GYN with difficulty in vaginal intercourse. She describes painful intercourse, and says that her vagina is too small. Her family is originally from Nigeria and her parents had nine children, all girls, three of which are in their 30s and unable to have children. Her sisters are unwilling to discuss their infertility, although she describes them as phenotypic females. Ms. Bamidele does not remember having a menstrual period, but did not seek medical care as she felt fine. At the age of 19, her gynecologist could not identify a cervix, and transabdominal ultrasound did not reveal the presence of uterus. She was told that she can never have children, but her parents did not want to pursue further evaluation, believing that everything would be fine. Her current physical examination was significant for scant axillary hair, normal breast development, normal labia and clitoris, with a short vaginal length of 5 cm and absence of cervix. Bimanual exam could not palpate a uterus. Although her major complaint was difficult intercourse, she wondered why she could not have children. What investigation would you pursue in order to make the diagnosis?

Disorders of sexual differentiation raise questions involving the multiple components of sexuality. Various related terms and definitions have become part of medical vocabulary.

Biological sex refers to an individual's intrinsic biological status as male or female based on karyotype, internal reproductive organs, and external genitalia. Often, the first question that expectant parents want to discuss is whether their child will be a boy or a girl. Biological sex disorders can present *in utero*. If so, they are usually detected when there is a discrepancy between karyotype and observed external genitalia. One subset of sex disorders will present at birth with ambiguous genitalia, and some represent true emergencies, such as salt-wasting congenital adrenal hyperplasia. Another subset of sex differentiation disorders are not diagnosed until adulthood. Both sex-linked and autosomal genes govern sexual differentiation.

It is important to understand that biological sex does influence gender and gender identity. **Gender** refers to the attitudes, feelings, and behaviors that a given culture associates with a person's biological sex, while **gender identity** refers to whether one identifies as being male, female, or transgender. A conflict between gender identity and biological sex may lead the individual to identify as transsexual.

Sexual orientation refers to the sex of those to whom one is sexually and romantically attracted. Gay men and lesbians are attracted to members of their own biological sex, heterosexuals are attracted to members of the other sex, and bisexuals are attracted to members of both sexes. Although we see sexual orientation in black and white terms, it can also be part of a continuum, and may differ at various stages of one's life. For example, some people may experience bisexual relationships for a time and then commit to either a homosexual or heterosexual orientation.

■ ORIGINS OF BIOLOGICAL SEX

Biological sex is closely intertwined with the biology and genesis of male and female gonads. Experiments in rabbits have shown that removal of either ovaries or testes will lead to the development of external genitalia consistent with female sex.[1] These experiments have been used to argue that ovarian development happens by default, while testes development requires the activation of genes that will lead to a male phenotype. This misconception has led to much research effort on male sex determination, but little is known regarding the pathways that lead to female sexual differentiation (Figure 13-1). Many genes are involved in the genesis of mammalian gonads and sex determination. It is of interest that, in some organisms, such as alligators and clownfish, environmental temperature and behavior play a dominant role in determining sex.[2]

Gonadal development is dependent on germ cells that are set aside early in the embryo. The germ cells are initially called primordial germ cells and migrate to

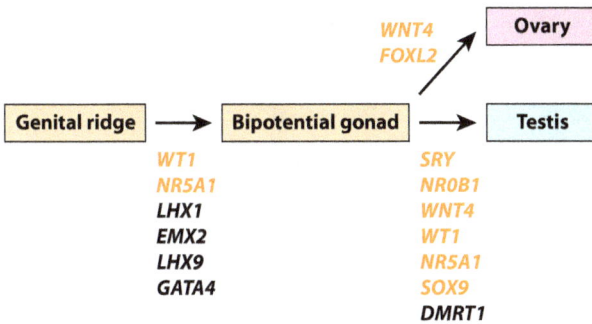

FIGURE 13-1. **Genes that orchestrate sex determination.** Many genes are known to play important functions for proper sexual differentiation to occur after primordial germ cells migrate to the genital ridge. The formation of the bipotential gonad requires a number of transcriptional regulators such as *WT1*, *NR5A1*, *LHX1*, *EMX2*, *LHX9*, and *GATA4*. *SRY*, *NR0B1*, *WNT4*, *SOX9*, *DMRT1*, *WT1*, and *NR5A1* genes drive the transition from bipotential gonad to testes. Little is known about genes that lead to ovarian development. Only two genes have been implicated in ovarian development: *WNT4* and *FOXL2*. *WT1*-Wilms tumor 1 gene, *NR5A1*- nuclear receptor subfamily 5, group A, member 1 gene, *LHX1*-LIM homeobox protein 1 gene, *EMX2*-empty spiracles homeobox 2 gene, *LHX9*-LIM homeobox protein 9 gene, *GATA4*-GATA binding protein 4 gene, *SRY*-sex determining region of Chr Y gene, *NR0B1*-nuclear receptor subfamily 0, group B, member 1 gene, *WNT4*-wingless-related MMTV integration site 4 gene, *SOX9*-SRY-box containing gene 9 gene, *DMRT1*-doublesex and mab-3 related transcription factor 1 gene, *FOXL2*-forkhead box L2 gene. Genes highlighted in orange are involved in human disorders of sexual differentiation.

the gonadal ridge where they divide by mitosis. The gonadal ridge will eventually become the gonad, either male or female. In the female, oocytes enter meiosis I, and arrest *in utero* in the diplotene stage, while male germ cells, called spermatogonia, do not enter meiosis until the onset of puberty.

Historically, the emphasis has been to elucidate the role of the Y chromosome in gonadal development and sex determination, as males are 46, XY and females are 46,XX. Since random X inactivation in females renders one X inactive in each cell, the Y chromosome must carry the determinant for testis development. It has been known since 1959 that the Y chromosome carries a determinant for testis development, and subsequent studies have shown that the *SRY* (sex-determining region of chromosome Y, also known as testis-determining factor or TDF) gene is essential for testis development.[3] However, the X chromosome is rich in genes necessary for testis development, and genetic defects on the X will cause abnormal male gonadal development. Both X chromosomes are essential in females for normal ovarian differentiation, and individuals with monosomy X (Turner syndrome) fail to develop normal ovaries.

Although emphasis was initially placed on the role of the sex chromosomes in sex determination, we now know that a number of autosomal genes are essential drivers of sexual differentiation. These include WT1 (Wilms tumor 1), NR0B1 (also known as steroidogenic factor 1), WNT4 (wingless-related MMTV integration site 4), SOX9, and DMRT1, among others. We also know that other, yet-to-be-discovered, autosomal genes for sex determination exist. The use of animal models such as transgenic mice has given us a good sense of the hierarchy of

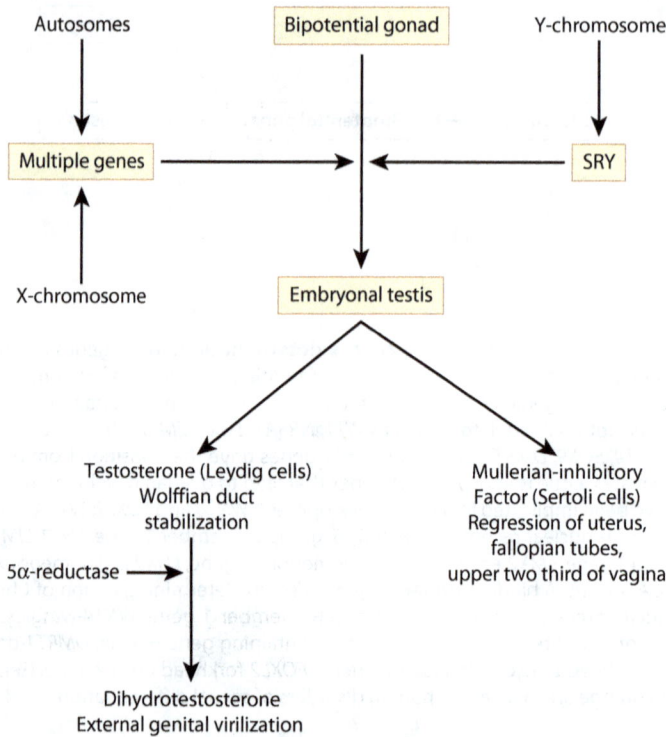

FIGURE 13-2. Simplified outline of the normal progression from the bipotential gonad to testis development and male internal and external genitalia.

genetic control of gonadal and sexual development[2] (Figure 13-1). Disorders in any of these genes can lead to ambiguous genitalia and sex reversal.

Figures 13-2 and 13-3 give a simplified outline of the progression from the bipotential gonad to the development of a functional ovary and testis and the resultant internal and external genitalia. As will be outlined in this chapter, many genes contribute to gonadal and sexual development, but understanding this basic framework helps in predicting the expected phenotype of a specific genetic mutation.

■ 46,XY DISORDERS OF SEXUAL DIFFERENTIATION

46,XY Gonadal Dysgenesis

In mammals, the gonads in both sexes have the potential to develop into either ovaries or testes. Normal male sexual differentiation in 46,XY individuals depends on the proper function and complex interaction of numerous testis-determining genes, including SRY, SOX9, NR5A1/SF1, NR0B1, AR, DHH, and CBX2.[4] Failure in the normal male sex differentiation process can cause complete or partial 46,XY gonadal dysgenesis.

Partial 46,XY gonadal dysgenesis is characterized by impaired testicular development and ambiguous external genitalia, including mild to severe penoscrotal

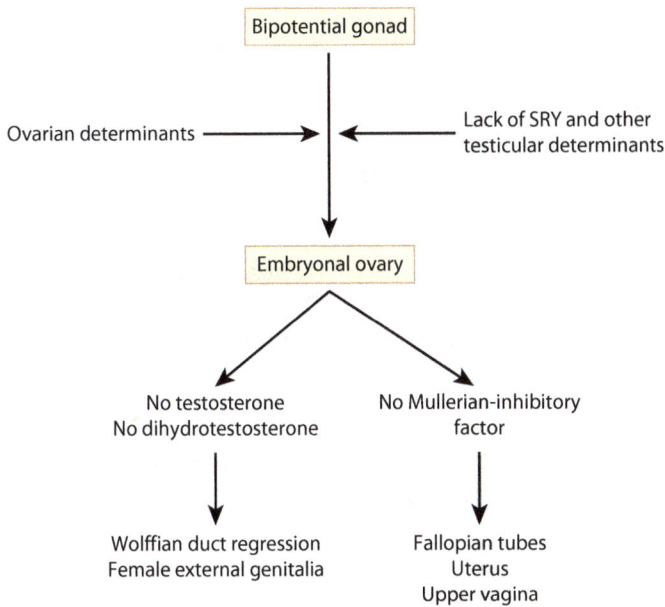

FIGURE 13-3. Simplified outline of the normal progression from the bipotential gonad to ovarian development and female internal and external genitalia.

hypospadias, dysgenetic (abnormally developed) testes, and reduced sperm production or none at all. Mullerian structures (uterus and fallopian tubes) may or may not be present.

Individuals with complete 46,XY gonadal dysgenesis, or Swyer syndrome, have normal female external genitalia and internal organs, but also have bilateral streak gonads.[5,6] Swyer syndrome has been estimated to occur in approximately 1 out of 30,000 individuals. Affected individuals are typically tall, lack secondary sexual characteristics, may have mild clitoromegaly, and are infertile. This condition commonly remains undiagnosed until adolescence, when puberty fails to occur. These females with a 46,XY karyotype have an increased risk of developing gonadoblastoma or dysgerminoma; therefore, the streak gonads are usually removed shortly after diagnosis. Women with Swyer syndrome cannot produce eggs; however, successful spregnancies have been achieved in some patients using donated eggs or embryos.

Complete 46,XY gonadal dysgenesis is a heterogeneous condition that may result from either chromosomal abnormalities (deletions, duplications, structural rearrangements) or point mutations in genes implicated in sexual differentiation. Despite considerable advances in understanding the genetic factors involved in gonadal determination and differentiation, a molecular diagnosis is made only in approximately 25% of cases with complete 46,XY gonadal dysgenesis. Mutations and deletions of the *SRY* gene are the cause of complete 46,XY gonadal dysgenesis in approximately 10% to 15% of patients with Swyer syndrome. The *SRY* gene is located on the short arm of the Y chromosome, and structural Y chromosome rearrangements resulting in the loss of the *SRY* gene include Yp deletions, dicentric Y isochromosomes composed of the long arms only, ring Y chromosomes, and Y-autosome translocations. Structurally abnormal Y chromosomes can be detected by conventional G-band chromosome analysis in some cases. However, molecular cytogenetic studies, such as fluorescence in situ hybridization (FISH) and array comparative genomic hybridization (aCGH) analyses, are essential for accurate diagnosis.[5]

Gene abnormalities on the X chromosome can result in 46,XY gonadal dysgenesis. X-chromosomal rearrangements in 46,XY females have led to the identification of a dosage-sensitive sex locus at the Xp21 region containing the *NR0B1* (also known as *DAX1*) gene. Patients with cytogenetically visible Xp21 duplications, containing many genes in addition to *NR0B1*, have a complex phenotype with congenital anomalies, dysmorphic features, intellectual disabilities, and gonadal dysgenesis. A submicroscopic 257-kb deletion upstream of *NR0B1* has been described in a 46,XY female with primary amenorrhea and gonadal dysgenesis.[7] This deletion probably affects regulatory sequences, leading to altered *NR0B1* expression and 46,XY gonadal dysgenesis consistent with *NR0B1* duplication.

Many autosomal genes are also implicated in disorders of sexual development in humans. Cytogenetically visible chromosome abnormalities, including deletions of 9p22-qter, 9q33, 10q25, 11p13, 13q32-q34, and 17q24, duplication of 1p34, and balanced translocations involving 17q24 have been identified in patients with XY gonadal dysgenesis. These rearrangements involve multiple genes and usually are associated with multiple congenital anomalies and intellectual disabilities (syndromic XY gonadal dysgenesis).[8] Isolated or nonsyndromic forms of XY gonadal dysgenesis are probably due to a single gene defect not detectable by a classical karyotype. Small deletions and duplications, encompassing a single gene, may be diagnosed using a high-resolution genome analysis technique such as aCGH (see Chapter 15).[8] Table 13-1 summarizes several genes that are known

■ **TABLE 13-1.** Genomic Imbalances Associated With Complete Gonadal Dysgenesis (CGD) in 46,XY Females

Locus	Genomic Abnormality	Gene	Molecular Mechanism	OMIM
1p36.12	Duplication	WNT4	Gain of function	603490
5q11.2	Deletion	MAP3K1	Loss of function	613762
8p23.1	Deletion downstream	GATA4	Regulatory region	600576
9p24.3	Deletion	DMRT1, DMRT2	Loss of function	154230
9q33.3	Deletion	NR5A1/SF1	Loss of function	612965
12q13.1	Homozygous deletion	DHH	Loss of function	233420
17q24	Translocation deletion	SOX9	Loss of function	
Xp21	Duplication deletion upstream	NR0B1/DAX1	Gain of function Regulatory region	300018
Yp11.31	Deletion	SRY	Loss-of-function	400044

to cause nonsyndromic XY gonadal dysgenesis, including those with microdeletions or microduplications affecting the gene or its regulatory regions. Using high-resolution whole genome and sex chromosome aCGH analyses, the cause of 46,XY gonadal dysgenesis can be elucidated in up to 30% of affected individuals, while the remaining patients may benefit from whole exome/genome sequencing tests.

Autosomal dominant mutations in the *WT1* gene (chromosome 11p13) cause the rare **Denys-Drash and Frasier syndromes**, with a phenotypic spectrum that includes 46,XY gonadal dysgenesis, gonadoblastomas, nephropathy, and renal tumors (Wilms tumor). Individuals with these syndromes may be born with genitalia that are ambiguous or with normal female external genitalia.

SOX9 is another autosomal gene important in sexual differentiation. Autosomal dominant mutations in *SOX9* cause a syndrome known as campomelic dysplasia. **Campomelic dysplasia** is characterized by ambiguous genitalia with bone abnormalities such as limb bowing and talipes equinovarus (club foot). Internal reproductive organs may be male (testes), female (ovaries), or a combination of the two. Most affected individuals are due to *de novo* mutations, but germline mosaicism in a parent accounts for the cases of recurrence within a family.

Persistent Mullerian duct syndrome is caused by autosomal recessive mutations within the anti-Mullerian hormone (AMH) gene or its receptor (AMHR) gene. These individuals present as 46,XY males with normal external genitalia, bilateral cryptorchidism and inguinal hernias, and an abnormal internal reproductive tract. An infantile uterus and fallopian tubes are usually identified by imaging studies, or at the time of hernia repair. AMH is secreted by the Sertoli cells in the male gonad and causes regression of the Mullerian ducts (uterus, fallopian tubes, cervix, and the upper two-third of the vagina) (Figure 13-2). Defective AMH signaling causes Mullerian ducts to persist. Testes are present in these individuals, but their fertility may be compromised due to associated abnormalities in the development of epididymis and vas deferens.

Androgen Insensitivity Syndrome

The androgen receptor is located on the X chromosome, and mutations in this receptor are X-linked recessive. Many mutations have been identified in the androgen receptor, and different mutations may have different effects on the receptor activity and its ability to transduce androgen signaling. Female (ie, XX) carriers of these mutations are usually unaffected. Total disruption of androgen receptor signaling in the male will cause complete androgen insensitivity syndrome as cells will be unable to respond to testosterone.

46,XY individuals having complete androgen insensitivity present with normal-appearing female external genitalia, without fallopian tubes or uterus, a blind-ending and short vagina, and bilateral testes. Because these individuals are phenotypically normal females at birth, they are not diagnosed until puberty when lack of menstruation and absent or decreased axillary and body hair causes concern. Breast development is usually normal, unlike Swyer syndrome. The testes can be located intra-abdominally at the internal inguinal ring, or herniate into the labia majora. Gonadal neoplasia occurs in approximately 2% to 5% of cases.

In partial androgen insensitivity, androgen receptor signaling is not completely abolished, and a variety of abnormalities might be seen, including hypospadias, clitoral hypertrophy, incomplete labial fusion, and ambiguous genitalia. A family history might help to determine the correct diagnosis, as could gene mutation analysis of the androgen receptor, or evidence of abnormal androgen binding in fibroblasts derived from genital skin.

5α-Reductase Deficiency

Conversion of testosterone to 5α-dihydrotesterone (DHT) requires the 5α-reductase enzyme. DHT is a potent androgen that is involved in the development of male external genitalia *in utero*. Autosomal recessive deficiency of 5α-reductase only affects genetic males because DHT has no known role during female development. Males with 5α-reductase deficiency can have male, female, or ambigous external genitalia. This range of phenotypes is related to the degree of 5α-reductase activity remaining in the mutant enzyme. Testes and Wolffian structures develop due to the presence of an intact Y chromosome, but these individuals usually have female external characteristics (Figure 13-2). They are usually raised as girls, but may have a male gender identity at the time of puberty, when virilization, hirsutism, deepening of the voice and enlargement of clitoris may occur. The pubertal androgenization is due to the increased presence of DHT secondary to the higher levels of testosterone being produced by the testes, and to partial activity of 5α-reductase enzyme allowing some conversion to DHT.

45,X/46,XY Mosaicism

The 45,X/46,XY karyotype is a relatively rare condition, occurring in approximately 1:15,000 live births. A spectrum of phenotypes has been reported ranging from females with Turner syndrome-like stigmata to phenotypically normal males with varying degrees of genital ambiguity.[9] Streak ovaries (ovaries replaced by fibrous tissue), ovotestis, and testes lacking germ cells (Sertoli cell-only syndrome) have been identified in such individuals. The diagnosis is usually made incidentally after a chromosome analysis for various other anomalies, such as ambiguous genitalia in a newborn, short stature and delayed puberty in an adolescent, infertility, or lack of virilization in adulthood. Most of these individuals will have abnormal gonadal histology, with a risk of gonadal malignancy approaching 15% (gonadectomy will need to be discussed). However, when diagnosed *in utero*, as a result of chorionic villus sampling and/or amniocentesis, 95% of these cases will show normal male external genitalia at the time of birth.[10]

■ 46,XX DISORDERS OF SEXUAL DIFFERENTIATION

46,XX Male Syndrome or Testicular Disorder of Sex Development

The XX male syndrome is a rare condition, with a frequency of 1:25,000 male newborns, and is characterized by the presence of a 46,XX karyotype, male and/or ambiguous genitalia, two testes, azoospermia (no sperm in the ejaculate) and absence of Mullerian structures.[4] Approximately 20% of boys with testicular disorder of sex development have ambiguous genitalia at birth, whereas the remaining 80% present with steroidogenic and spermatogenic dysfunction after puberty.

The majority of males with the 46,XX karyotype are found to be *SRY*-positive by either FISH or polymerase chain reaction amplification.[4,11] In most instances, 46,XX male syndrome is caused by an exchange of segments between the short arms of the X and Y chromosomes (X;Y translocation) during paternal meiosis (Figure 13-4A),

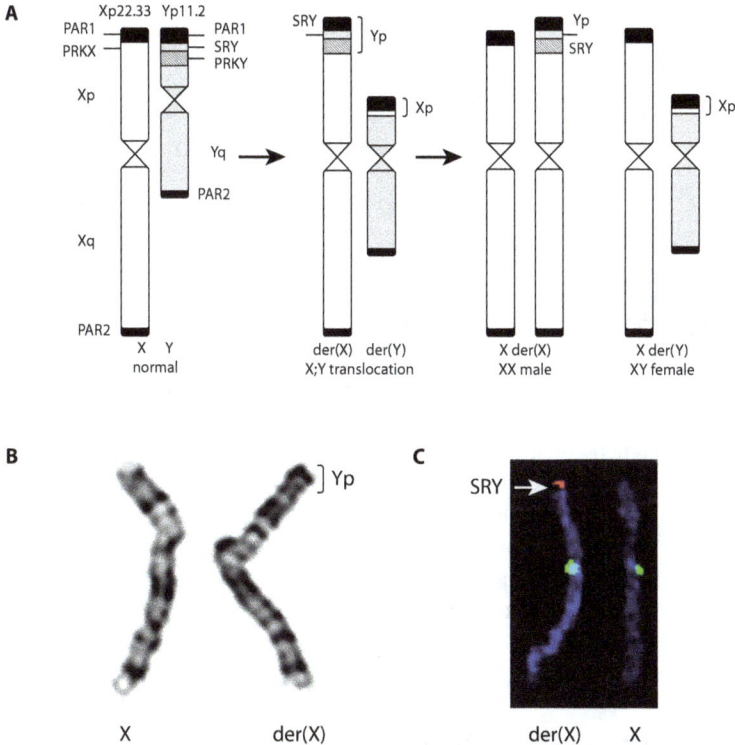

FIGURE 13-4. X-Y chromosomes translocation. (A) During male meiosis, X and Y chromosomes normally pair and recombine within the two homologous regions (pseudoautosomal regions, PAR1 and PAR2) located at the distal short and long arms of sex chromosomes. Aberrant recombination involving highly homologous DNA sequences such as the *PRKX* and *PRKY* genes, results in exchange of X-specific and Y-specific DNA segments. The X-Y translocation causes transposition of the *SRY* gene from Y to X chromosome resulting in derivative chromosome X (derX) containing *SRY*, and derivative chromosome Y (derY), deleted for the *SRY* gene. Fertilization by a sperm containing the derivative X chromosome will conceive an *SRY*-positive XX male, whereas sperm carrying derivative Y chromosome, deleted for *SRY*, will conceive an XY female. (B) Partial karyotype and (C) fluorescence in situ hybridization (FISH) analysis in the XX-male. (B) Chromosome analysis detected a derivative chromosome X containing the Yp segment at the distal short arm of X chromosome. (C) FISH analysis with *SRY*-specific probe (red signal, arrow) shows that *SRY* gene is present in the derivative X chromosome. Centromere of the X chromosome is labeled in green.

■ **TABLE 13-2.** Genomic Imbalances Associated With Complete Gonadal Dysgenesis (CGD) in 46,XX Males

Locus	Genomic Abnormality	Gene	Molecular Mechanism	Phenotype	OMIM
1p34.3	Duplication	RSPO1	Gain-of function	CGD, palmoplantar hyperkeratosis	610644
17q24	Duplication downstream	regulatory region SOX9	Gain-of function	CGD	613080
Xq26	Duplication deletion upstream	SOX3, regulatory region	Gain-of function	CGD	300833
Yp11	Presence	SRY	X-Y or Yp-autosome translocation	CGD	400044

resulting in the derivative chromosome X containing the *SRY* gene (Figure 13-4B, C), and the derivative chromosome Y deleted for *SRY*. Fertilization with an abnormal gamete containing either the *SRY*-positive X chromosome or the Y chromosome with the *SRY* gene deletion will result in a sterile XX male or XY female, respectively. Translocations between the Y and autosomal chromosomes can also give rise to *SRY*-positive XX males, where the *SRY* gene is located on the autosomal chromosome.

About 10% of 46,XX men are *SRY*-negative and can present with either ambiguous genitalia or normal male genitalia at birth.[12] *SRY* normally triggers testes formation by activating expression of *SOX9*, located at 17q24.3. Like *SRY*, *SOX9* is necessary for testis differentiation, and its overexpression can lead to male development in the absence of *SRY*. Table 13-2 outlines several examples of genomic imbalance that result in 46,XX males.

Congenital Adrenal Hyperplasia

Congenital adrenal hyperplasia (CAH) is an autosomal recessive disorder caused by defects in the synthesis of cortisol from cholesterol in the adrenal cortex. The most common cause of CAH is deficiency of the 21-hydoxylase enzyme *(CYP21A2)*. It affects approximately 1:15,000 individuals in the United States. 21-Hydroxylase deficiency causes excessive adrenal androgen biosynthesis and virilization of affected females. A subset of newborns will have a life-threatening salt-wasting form of CAH. Virilized females usually present with ambiguous external genitalia and a normal uterus and ovaries. Males with 21-hydroxylase deficiency do not have ambiguous genitalia, but will suffer from cortisol and mineralocorticoid deficiency.

The diagnosis of CAH is established by the finding of highly elevated levels of the 17-hydroxyprogesterone, a precursor to cortisol, and by molecular genetic testing for mutations in the *CYP21A2* gene. Classical 21-hydroxylase deficiency is a life-threatening disorder that requires prompt neonatal diagnosis and intervention to replace cortisol and mineralocorticoids.

A nonclassical form of 21-hydroxylase deficiency is a relatively common autosomal recessive disorder, with an incidence of 1:100, that can present with hyperandrogenic symptoms, including advanced bone age, early pubic hair, precocious puberty, tall stature, infertility, hirsutism, polycystic ovaries, and irregular menstrual periods in women.

Measurement of 17-hydroxyprogesterone, androstenedione, cortisone, and aldosterone levels and performance of an ACTH stimulation test to determine the degree of 17-hydroxyprogesterone rise above baseline can distinguish individuals with classical and nonclassical forms. Individuals with nonclassical 21-hydroxylase deficiency may be at risk to have a child with the classical form of CAH. Preconception counseling for individuals affected by the nonclassical form of CAH, and carrier testing of their partners should be offered in order to diagnose early, and manage, infants at risk for 21-hydroxylase deficiency.

A less common form of congenital adrenal hyperplasia involves recessive mutations in the 11β-hydroxylase gene, *CYP11B1*. The 11β-hydroxylase deficiency presents with ambiguous genitalia, but differs from 21-hydroxylase deficiency in that both males and females present with hypertension and elevated levels of deoxycortisol and deoxycorticosterone. The 11β-hydroxylase deficiency is a rare disorder, affecting approximately 1:100,000 live births.

Aromatase Deficiency

Aromatase is an enzyme, encoded by the *CYP19A1* gene, that converts androgens into estradiol. Autosomal recessive mutations in *CYP19A1* lead to aromatase deficiency, hypoestrogenism, and elevated levels of androgens. This is a rare disorder, affecting fewer than one in a million newborns. Females born with aromatase deficiency often have clitoral hypertrophy, tend to be taller due to delayed epiphyseal closure, fail to develop breasts, and do not menstruate (primary amenorrhea). These individuals are characterized by hypergonadotropic (elevated luteinizing and follicle stimulating hormone levels) hypogonadism. Interestingly, mothers carrying affected individuals develop hirsutism and acne due to fetal aromatase deficiency. Maternal virilization reverses after delivery of the affected fetus and placenta. In affected fetuses, the fetal dehydroepiandrosterone sulfate cannot be converted to estrogen by the placenta, and is converted to testosterone peripherally, causing the maternal symptoms. Affected males do not present with obvious defects at birth, but present later with tall stature due to delayed epiphyseal closure. Estrogen replacement therapy reverses the symptoms in both males and females.

■ PRACTICAL CONSIDERATIONS

Disorders of sexual differentiation represent a medical emergency, and usually involve a multidisciplinary team to diagnose and manage the affected individual. The diagnosis may begin *in utero*, when ultrasound examination detects ambiguous genitalia or when a discrepancy between genetic sex and phenotypic sex is determined by chorionic villus sampling or amniocentesis. If ambiguous genitalia are suspected on prenatal ultrasound, a three-generation pedigree should be elicited to uncover any history of structural birth defects or disorders of sexual differentiation. Maternal health and drug exposure should be documented. It is also important to assess fetal growth, and whether additional structural birth defects are present.

Amniocentesis (if not already done) should be discussed to determine the genetic sex of the baby, and a portion of the liquor saved, should additional tests prove necessary. If the karyotype returns as 46,XX, the most likely diagnosis is congenital adrenal hyperplasia, and amniotic fluid 17-hydroxyprogesterone levels should be measured. If high levels of 17-hydroxyprogesterone are present, the diagnosis is probably 21-hydroxylase deficiency. Pediatric endocrinology and neonatology should be involved prenatally to assist in the diagnosis and to plan for postnatal care to prevent complications related to the life-threatening salt-wasting variety of 21-hydroxylase deficiency.

If amniocentesis shows a 46,XY karyotype, the differential is much broader, and a specific diagnosis may be possible in only 25% of cases. Mutations or deletions studies for the *SRY* gene should be done in such cases.

In the vignette at the beginning of the chapter, Ms. Bamidele's disorder would not have been detected prenatally, or on the postnatal newborn exam. It is important, first, to determine the karyotype. In her case, she is a genetic male, 46,XY, with normal female external genitalia and well-developed breasts. *SRY* studies were done to assess for a *SRY* gene deletion or deleterious mutations, and *SRY* was present. The presence of *SRY* and well-developed breasts rules out Swyer syndrome, and would be consistent with complete androgen insensitivity syndrome. A family history of nine girls, three of whom are infertile, and no boys is also consistent with an X-linked recessive disorder of sex differentiation. Androgen receptor gene sequencing was done and identified an inactivating mutation, confirming the diagnosis of complete androgen insensitivity syndrome. Her three infertile sisters may also be genetic males with the same mutation in the androgen receptor gene as Ms. Bamidele.

Many cases of 46,XY sex reversal and ambiguous genitalia remain unsolved. We expect that the future development of whole exome sequencing to comprehensively analyze many of the genes responsible for disorders of sexual differentiation should substantially increase the diagnostic yield and will lead to discoveries of novel genetic mechanisms.

REFERENCES

1. Jost A. Hormonal factors in the sex differentiation of the mammalian foetus. *Philos Trans R SocLond B Biol Sci.* 1970;259(828):119-130.
2. Wilhelm D, Palmer S, Koopman P. Sex determination and gonadal development in mammals. *Physiol Rev.* 2007;87:1-28.

3. Berta P, Hawkins JB, Sinclair AH, et al. Genetic evidence equating *SRY* and the testis-determining factor. *Nature.* 1990;348:448-450.

4. Kousta E, Papathanasiou A, Skordis N. Sex determination and disorders of sex development according to the revised nomenclature and classification in 46,XX individuals. *Hormones (Athens).* 2010;9:218-131.

5. Simpson JL, Rajkovic A. Ovarian differentiation and gonadal failure. *Am J Med Genet.* 1999;89:186-200.

6. Jorgensen PB, Kjartansdottir KR, Fedder J. Care of women with XY karyotype: a clinical practice guideline. *Fertil Steril.* 2010;94:105-113.

7. Smyk M, Berg JS, Pursley A, et al. Male-to-female sex reversal associated with an ~250 kb deletion upstream of *NR0B1* (DAX1). *Hum Genet.* 2007;122:63-70.

8. Rajcan-Separovic E. Chromosome microarrays in human reproduction. *Hum Reprod Update.* 2012;18:555-567.

9. Johansen ML, Hagen CP, Meyts, ERD, etc. 45,X/46,XY mosaicism: phenotypic characteristics, growth, and reproductive function—a retrospective longitudinal study. *J Clin Endocrinol. Metab.* 2012;97:E1540-E1549.

10. Chang HJ, Clark RD, Bachman H. The phenotype of 45,X/46,XY mosaicism: an analysis of 92 prenatally diagnosed cases. *Am J Hum Genet.* 1990;46:156-167.

11. Turek PJ. Practical approaches to the diagnosis and management of male infertility. *Nat Clin Pract Urol.* 2005;2:226-238.

12. Vetro A, Ciccone R, Giorda R. XX males SRY negative: a confirmed cause of infertility. *J Med Genet.* 2011;48:710-712.

Genetics of Infertility and Pregnancy Loss

Case 1: John is a 35-year-old executive of a manufacturing company who presented with infertility. He and his wife have had unprotected intercourse over the past 18 months and have not been able to conceive. John has known that he had small testes since college following a regular physical exam. He denies any childhood problems or developmental delay. He does not recollect being different from other boys around puberty. He did grow rapidly, with a height of 5 ft in 4th grade, and 6 ft in 6th grade. He is currently 6 ft 5 inches tall. He has noticed difficulty with erection and libido since age 30 and thought it was normal. He currently has a low libido and at times difficulty in achieving orgasm. His semen analysis 2 months ago revealed azoospermia. What additional testing would you recommend for John?

Infertility is defined as a failure to conceive after 12 months of unprotected intercourse[1-3] and it affects 10% to 15% of American couples. Infertility is a devastating disorder that affects equally men and women, and both male and female evaluations are necessary to optimize a couple's success for conception. Infertility can be syndromic, ie, expressed as part of a major genetic syndrome, or idiopathic, where the cause is unknown and usually confined to the gonads with no obvious extra-gonadal manifestation. A three-generation family pedigree is very helpful in detecting clues to heritable disorders. For example, a family history of infertility and anemia or cancer may indicate Fanconi syndrome, while a family history with infertility in the females and mental retardation among males may indicate the Fragile X syndrome. A detailed physical examination is important to rule out dysmorphic features, which may be an indication of syndromic cause of infertility.

■ MALE INFERTILITY

The causes of male infertility include environmental exposures, anatomic obstruction, and genetic, infectious, and autoimmune disorders and other diverse etiologies.[1] Male infertility has many psychological, economic, and social sequelae, including decreased quality of life, and can be associated with serious medical disorders.[1,12]

Among infertile men, almost 20% have azoospermia (no sperm in the ejaculate) or oligozoospermia/oligospermia (low-sperm concentration, less than 15 million sperm per milliliter of ejaculate), while another 20% have asthenospermia (sperm with low motility). Other sperm abnormalities include teratozoospermia (abnormal sperm morphology). Genetic factors are known to play an important role in male infertility, and at least 2300 testes genes may be involved in male fertility.

■ CHROMOSOMAL CAUSES OF MALE INFERTILITY

Studies in infertile men demonstrated that up to 20% carry constitutional chromosome aberrations.[4,5] Genomic aberrations found in these patients include numerical abnormalities, such as Klinefelter syndrome and its variants; XYY karyotype; testicular disorders of sex development, such as XX males; structural chromosome rearrangements, including Robertsonian translocations, balanced reciprocal translocations and inversions; as well as submicroscopic DNA copy number alterations (microdeletions and microduplications) encompassing genes associated with spermatogenesis or gonadal development.

Klinefelter Syndrome

Klinefelter men can present with variable phenotypes and the only reliable diagnosis is based on the karyotype. These men usually present due to infertility and nonobstructive azoospermia. Physical examination is significant for small testes. Other findings that have been associated with Klinefelter men, but are not always present, include gynecomastia, long legs/arms, developmental delay, speech and language deficits, learning disabilities and inferior performance in school. Serum testosterone levels may be low with elevated follicle stimulating hormone and luteinizing hormone levels. Klinefelter syndrome occurs in approximately 0.1% of live male births and is the most common chromosomal aberration among infertile men, accounting for 14% of azoospermia patients.[6] Klinefelter syndrome is characterized by the presence of one or more extra X chromosomes in association with a normal Y chromosome. The most common variant, the 47,XXY karyotype, is seen in approximately 90% of Klinefelter men.

Due to the variability of the phenotype, Klinefelter syndrome is underdiagnosed, with only 10% of Klinefelter patients recognized prepubertally and an additional 15% identified after puberty.[4,5,7] Infertility and small testes are the most prevalent characteristics in adult Klinefelter syndrome patients. The testes in adult Klinefelter syndrome males are characterized by extensive fibrosis and hyalinization of the seminiferous tubules and impaired spermatogenesis, with azoospermia or severe oligozoospermia. Although most Klinefelter syndrome patients are infertile, testicular spermatozoa can be identified and recovered from at least 50% of men with the nonmosaic 47,XXY karyotype.[4,8] Testicular sperm extraction (TESE) combined with intracytoplasmic sperm injection (ICSI) allows some patients with Klinefelter syndrome to father their own biological children.[6,9]

Sperm from Klinefelter syndrome men usually have a normal 23,X or 23,Y haploid chromosome complement. Despite this, an increased frequency for both autosomal and sex chromosome aneuploidy has been reported in fetuses of such men.[4,10]

Y Chromosome Microdeletions

The human Y chromosome contains many genes that are essential for male sex determination and spermatogenesis.[1,11] Microdeletions (deletions that cannot be visualized via standard microscopy) on the long arm of chromosome Y (Yq) are one of the most significant pathogenic defects in infertile males, found in about 10% of men with oligozoospermia, and in up to 15% of azoospermic patients.[5,6,8] The most common deletions involve the AZF region that is made up of three genetic domains (AZFa, AZFb, and AZFc) located on the long arm of the Y chromosome. Microdeletions encompassing genes other than those located in the AZFa, AZFb, and AZFc regions on the Y chromosome have been proposed to influence spermatogenesis, although their role remains to be elucidated. In addition, gross structural abnormalities of the Yq chromosome, such as whole long arm deletions (del(Y)(q11.2)), isochromosome Yp (i(Yp)) and dicentric Yp (dic(Yp)), can result in complete absence of germ cells.[4,9] These abnormalities are much less common than the microdeletions.

Balanced Chromosome Rearrangements

Structural chromosomal abnormalities are frequent in infertile men, with an overall incidence of about 5%, tenfold higher than the 0.5% prevalence for structural chromosomal abnormalities in the general population.[6,12] Chromosome rearrangements are found in approximately 14% of azoospermic and 4.5% of oligozoospermic patients. Autosome aberrations (3%) are more commonly associated with oligozoospermia, whereas sex chromosome defects (12.6%) predominate among azoospermic men.[12,13] Structural chromosome rearrangements may cause impaired spermatogenesis by adversely affecting chromosome synapsis during meiosis.[5,13] Alternatively, chromosome breaks that cause rearrangements may result in disruption/inactivation of a single dosage-sensitive gene(s) involved in spermatogenesis, thus resulting in the arrest of normal male germ cell development.[12, 13]

Carriers of balanced chromosome rearrangements usually have a normal phenotype and are often diagnosed during evaluation of their infertility problem, or following the birth of a child with an unbalanced chromosome complement. Chromosome segregation analyses demonstrate a high proportion (up to 80%) of unbalanced spermatozoa among carriers of reciprocal translocations. Fertility problems in male carriers can be attributed to disturbance of the meiotic process, and various degrees of sperm defects. However, the presence of a balanced chromosome rearrangement is not necessarily associated with spermatogenic failure. Infertility and the finding of a balanced rearrangement should not preclude doing a full infertility evaluation on the couple. Fertilization by an unbalanced gamete does occur, and many resulting embryos do not survive. Therefore, individuals carrying balanced rearrangements can benefit from preimplantation genetic diagnosis (PGD) to identify and implant embryos with a normal or balanced chromosome complement.

Individuals who carry chromosome inversions are usually healthy; however, infertility, recurrent pregnancy losses, and chromosomally abnormal offspring have been reported.[5,12,13] In carriers of paracentric inversions (see Chapter 2), unbalanced chromosomal complements have been reported in about 1% of spermatozoa, but this finding is based on a limited number of individuals.[13] In contrast, carriers of pericentric inversions may have a high proportion (up to 54%) of spermatozoa with unbalanced recombinant chromosomes.[5,9] In general, large pericentric inversions (encompassing more than half of the chromosome length) are more likely to produce unbalanced chromosomes, and are therefore more frequently observed among infertile men.

Complex chromosome rearrangements (CCRs) involve at least three breakpoints and exchange of genetic material between two or more chromosomes, and occur in around 0.5% of newborns.[14] Unbalanced CCRs are often associated with intellectual disability and congenital abnormalities. Balanced CCRs are seen in phenotypically normal individuals with a history of recurrent abortions and infertility. Each CCR is unique and reproductive risks will depend upon multiple factors such as chromosome origin, location of breakpoints, number of chromosomes involved, genome content, and rearrangement type and complexity. There are 64 possible combinations of chromosomes in spermatozoa of a carrier for CCR with three breaks involving three chromosomes. The number of combinations increases with the involvement of additional chromosomes and/or breakpoints. Because of the low proportion of balanced sperm available (~10%-20%), intracytoplasmic sperm injection is not recommended in male CCR carriers.

Robertsonian translocations are the most common structural chromosomal rearrangement in humans, resulting in a derivative chromosome composed of the long arms of two acrocentric chromosomes (13, 14, 15, 21, and 22). The most frequent Robertsonian translocations are der(13;14) and der(14;21) with incidences of about 1:1000 and 1:5000, respectively.[15,16] Carriers of Robertsonian translocations have an increased risk for infertility, chromosomally unbalanced offspring, and spontaneous abortions, but are otherwise healthy. Studies involving male carriers of der(13;14) showed that in about 80% of cases the partners had spontaneous pregnancies, while in 20% of cases the male carriers were infertile.[15,16] Among infertile male patients, 1.6% are Robertsonian translocation carriers. The infertility in these individuals likely involves abnormal meiosis with subsequent meiotic arrest that causes oligozoospermia or azoospermia.

47,XYY Karyotype

An extra copy of the Y chromosome is present in 47,XYY males. This chromosomal aneuploidy occurs in 1 of 1000 live male births in the general population, and is seen more frequently in the infertile population. The vast majority of men with the 47,XYY karyotype have normal phenotype and normal fertility. Semen analyses in a minority of some men may show oligozoospermia or azoospermia, while the majority of 47,XYY males are fertile with normal semen parameters, and produce normal haploid spermatozoa.[9]

■ OBSTRUCTIVE AZOOSPERMIA

Cystic Fibrosis and Congenital Absence of Vas Deferens

Obstructive azoospermia is due to a physical obstruction between the testes and the urethra and can be caused by vasectomy, agenesis of the vas deferens, or ejaculatory duct obstruction among other things. Obstructive azoospermia can be differentiated from nonobstructive azoospermia by testicular biopsy. In obstructive azoospermia, testicular biopsy will show normal spermatogenesis, and such individuals are candidates for intracytoplasmic sperm injection (ICSI), while few if any sperm will be identified in nonobstructive azoospermia. Congenital absence of vas deferens is a form of obstructive azoospermia, and accounts for approximately 2% of all cases of male infertility, and up to 25% of cases of obstructive azoospermia. More than 95% of males with cystic fibrosis have congenital absence of vas deference (CAVD) bilaterally with resulting azoospermia. This has led to investigations whether men with isolated CAVD, but without overt symptoms of cystic fibrosis (pulmonary, pancreatic and intestinal manifestations), also carry mutations in the cystic fibrosis gene. Multiple studies have shown that the majority of men with CAVD do carry mutations in the cystic fibrosis gene. Approximately 80% of men with CAVD carry at least one mutation and approximately 50% carry two mutations. Mutations in the CFTR gene in the idiopathic form of CAVD are usually compound heterozygous and involve one allele that is highly damaging such as F508del, and mild alleles such as 5T (c.1210-12T[5]) and R117H (c.350G >A).

Men with CAVD should be offered genetic screening for CFTR mutations, and such couples should undergo genetic counseling. Men with CAVD are candidates for intracytoplasmic sperm injection, and at high risk for carrying a CFTR mutation. Hence, they are at risk to have a child with cystic fibrosis. If testing of the male with CAVD shows mutations in the CFTR gene, their partner should be tested for CFTR mutations prior to ICSI to establish her carrier status and provide appropriate risk assessment. Preimplantation genetic diagnosis can be offered to couples when both are carriers for CFTR mutations in order to identify which embryos are affected.

In Case 1, John had chromosome studies done, and the karyotype showed 47,XXY, consistent with the diagnosis of Klinefelter syndrome. Hormonal studies indicated low testosterone and elevated FSH levels, consistent with hypergonadotropic hypogonadism due to absence of germ cells and gonadal dysfunction. John and his wife are interested in further understanding the Klinefelter syndrome, and how it will affect their ability to conceive. Laura is currently 35 years of age and does not have children. This is a first marriage for both of them. John was counseled that his lifespan will be normal, and that the extra X chromosome results in decreased fertility due to unknown mechanisms. Because of germ cell and spermatogonia depletion in the Klinefelter syndrome, testosterone production is lowered with resultant decreased libido and sexual performance. John was initiated on testosterone replacement and noticed improvement with libido, erection, and memory after 2 months of treatment. He was referred to an urologist, who performed testicular biopsy to determine the presence of viable sperm. Testicular biopsy revealed complete absence of sperm and John and Laura were not candidates for intracytoplasmic sperm injection (ICSI). The couple was counseled to consider sperm from a donor, or adoption as options to have a child.

Case 2: Ellie, who is 17, and her parents came to the clinic to discuss the diagnosis of Turner syndrome. Ellie's mother stated that her pregnancy was unremarkable and Ellie weighed 6 lb and 6 oz at the time of birth. Ellie's mom denies noticing a webbed neck or swollen feet and extremities at the time of birth. They did not notice any problems with Ellie during her early development, but they did notice that she appeared to stop growing at age 12. She is currently 60 in (approx. 5th percentile). Lack of menarche prompted karyotype analysis that showed a chromosomal

mosaicism for 45,X in 90% of the cells, and 46,X with Xq isochromosome in 10% of the cells, consistent with Turner syndrome. Additional evaluations revealed normal cardiac anatomy on a suboptimal echocardiogram, normal renal ultrasound, lack of ovaries on the pelvic ultrasound, and an elevated TSH with borderline T4 levels. Ellie had a newborn hearing screen, which she passed according to her mother, but no recent audiometry has been done. Her physical exam was significant for short stature, Tanner stage II breast development (Tanner V expected at her age), normal pubic hair, small hands, with short thumbs, and a somewhat swollen appearance. Her feet appeared small, with a short penultimate toe on the right foot. How do you counsel Ellie and her parents?

■ FEMALE INFERTILITY

Female infertility is often due to impairment of ovarian function that can result from several different genetic mechanisms—numerical X chromosome abnormalities, including Turner syndrome and the triple X karyotype; balanced structural chromosomal rearrangements, genomic imbalances involving the X chromosome and autosomes, XY gonadal dysgenesis, and single gene alterations leading to ovarian dysgenesis, premature ovarian failure, and reproductive dysfunction. X chromosome-linked aberrations play a major role among currently known genetic defects.[17]

Premature ovarian insufficiency (POI), also called premature ovarian failure (POF), not caused by surgery, chemotherapy, radiation or other exposures such as chronic smoking, affects approximately 1% to 4% of women, and is clinically defined as a cessation of menses prior to age 40 (normal being 50-52), with elevated FSH levels and low serum estradiol levels.[18] The incidence of POI prior to age 30 is 0.1%. Women with POI present with amenorrhea, either primary or secondary, hot flashes, and vaginal dryness. Women with POI have 50% higher overall mortality, with an 80% increase in mortality due to ischemic heart disease, and an increased risk of cognitive impairment and dementia, as well as premature osteoporosis.[19-22] The association of POI with accelerated overall aging, signifies that ovarian aging may be a window into women's aging in general.

■ CHROMOSOME CAUSES OF FEMALE INFERTILITY

Turner Syndrome

Turner syndrome is a common genetic disorder that results from a loss of a sex chromosome (45,X or monosomy X) in a phenotypic female. Turner syndrome occurs in approximately 1 in 2000 to 3000 female live births as a result of mainly paternal (80%) chromosome nondisjunction during meiosis.[23] The vast majority of monosomy X conceptions are aborted, and only 1% to 3% of conceptions become viable and survive to birth. Clinical manifestations are variable in affected females, and include short stature, skeletal abnormalities, congenital heart and kidney anomalies, and characteristic physical features, such as a wide and webbed neck, a low hairline at the back of the neck, and absence of secondary sexual characteristics.[17] Individuals with Turner syndrome do not undergo puberty, and have infantile internal and external genitalia. Turner individuals are on average 20 cm (7.9 in) shorter than their adult peers. Early diagnosis is therefore important in order to initiate growth hormone therapy as early as possible. Growth hormone treatment can commence prior to age 4, and is unlikely to help after age 13. Transdermal estrogen replacement should be initiated around 13 years of age to allow normal pubertal and sexual development and prevent osteoporosis. Most women with Turner syndrome have normal intelligence, although cognitive deficits, developmental delays, nonverbal learning disabilities, and behavioral problems do occur. All girls with short stature should have chromosome studies to rule out Turner syndrome.

Approximately half of females diagnosed with Turner syndrome have 45,X chromosome complement. The other half are mosaic individuals where 45,X cells can occur either with normal 46,XX cells, with cells that have 46 chromosomes but one of the two X chromosomes is structurally abnormal, or with 46,XY cells.[17] The chromosome constitution and level of mosaicism influence the resulting phenotype in Turner syndrome individuals.

In Turner girls, primordial germ cells form but are lost rapidly, and hypoplastic "streak" gonads, composed of fibrous tissue, are detected at the time of puberty.[17] In females, one X chromosome in every cell is inactivated; however, gene expression from both X chromosomes in oocytes is necessary for normal ovarian development. Haploinsufficiency for the X-linked genes during critical times in ovarian development is likely responsible for gonadal dysgenesis that leads to infertility in 45,X individuals. The ovaries of teenage girls who have Turner syndrome with X chromosome mosaicism can contain follicles and a subset of Turner mosaic women experience menarche, spontaneous menstrual cycles and pregnancy.[17, 24]

A combination of a 45,X (Turner syndrome) cell line and a normal 46,XX chromosome complement is the most common form of mosaicism in Turner syndrome individuals. Many patients with mosaicism for monosomy X are mildly affected, undergo breast development, menstruate, and may present in clinic only due to infertility or premature ovarian insufficiency as a major concern. The risk for premature ovarian failure in mosaic Turner syndrome increases when mosaicism is greater than 10%. It is important to remember, however, that mosaicism in blood does not predict mosaicism within the ovary. It is therefore prudent to follow individuals with low-level mosaicism with yearly anti-mullerian hormone (AMH) levels as an indirect measure of ovarian reserves.

Ellie and her parents wanted to understand more about the consequences and management options. They understood that ovarian insufficiency occurs in most girls with Turner syndrome, and her pelvic ultrasound is consistent with ovarian insufficiency. Eggs form in girls with Turner syndrome, but few survive beyond puberty, leading to ovarian failure and inability to conceive. Without eggs, normal ovarian development does not occur and ovarian derived estrogen is not produced. Ellie was diagnosed relatively late and should be on appropriate estrogen replacement therapy until age 50. Bone mineral density should be assessed to rule out osteoporosis. Oocyte donation provides an option in the future to achieve pregnancy. However, pregnancy is a relative contraindication in women with Turner syndrome, due to the possibility of aortic dissection. Her recent echocardiogram was normal, but limited by inadequate visualization. The echocardiogram should be repeated in 5 years to assess aortic root dilatation. She is also at risk for hypothyroidism. Deafness is more common among Turner girls, and repeat audiometry is indicated now, and every 5 years. Moreover, she should have regular blood pressure check-ups, as Ellie is at risk for hypertension as well as diabetes. Because of her late diagnosis, she is not a candidate for growth hormone therapy.

47,XXX Karyotype

Trisomy X, triple X, or 47,XXX karyotype is caused by a nondisjunction event of the X chromosome, either during gametogenesis or after conception.[25] Trisomy X affects approximately 1/1000 girls. It is estimated that only 10% of cases are diagnosed, as a majority of these women are normal. Some women with 47,XXX can be taller than average, may present with learning disabilities, delayed development of motor skills, or speech and language problems. The vast majority of women with trisomy X syndrome have normal onset of puberty, normal sexual development, and normal fertility.[25] However, some individuals are not able to conceive due to premature ovarian insufficiency or genitourinary malformations. Trisomy X syndrome is found in approximately 3% of females with premature ovarian insufficiency.[25]

Trisomy X is of maternal origin in 90% of cases and of paternal origin in 10% of cases. Mosaicism is present in about 20% of cases and is caused by X chromosome nondisjunction during early embryo development. Phenotype and fertility in mosaic cases are adversely affected by the presence of abnormal cells such as 45,X (Turner) or 48,XXXX (tetrasomy X). Fertile females with trisomy X produce normal haploid gametes, with no increased risk for a 47,XXX or 47,XXY child.[25]

Case 3: Kelly is a 37-year-old woman who was referred for further management because she was found to carry a premutation for fragile X, with 64 CGG repeats identified in one of her FMR1 alleles. Kelly had a baby in 2008, breast fed for about 11 months, and did not have the period till about 8 to 9 months after her first delivery. For the past 2 years, her menstrual periods have been irregular with inter-menstrual intervals longer than 30 days, and skipping of some months. Kelly has not experienced hot flashes, night sweats, or vaginal dryness. She does complain of feeling irritable at times. She wants to conceive, but has been unable despite 12 months of unprotected intercourse. Her infertility work-up revealed a FSH of 56 mIU/mL, up from 37 mIU/mL 6 months ago. Her LH values were also elevated. She had a normal TSH and free T4. Her karyotype showed normal number and banding, except for inversion on chromosome 9 that is found in 2% of the population, and is considered a normal variant, 46,XX,inv(9)(p11q13). Kelly has a sister who is healthy and pregnant. Fragile X results are pending on Kelly's sister. Kelly's aunt on the maternal side has mild MR and another aunt has an "autistic" son.

Genes on the X Chromosome Implicated in Ovarian Failure

To date, the number and precise location of genes relevant to X-linked premature ovarian insufficiency are still under investigation. Despite a wealth of evidence implicating the X-chromosome and ovarian reserves, only the *FMR1* gene has reached clinical significance for its association with premature ovarian insufficiency.[17,24] Many clinics currently screen their patients for *FMR1* premutation status and the interpretation of such results is important in patient management. Within the 5′ untranslated region of the *FMR1* gene are CGG trinucleotide repeats. The number of CGG repeats is less than 55 in the normal individual. Individuals who carry between 55 and 200 repeats are called premutation carriers. The prevalence of premutation carriers is approximately 1/150. Men and women who are carriers for the premutation are at risk of developing fragile X-associated tremor and ataxia syndrome. Women who carry the premutation are at approximately 20% risk of developing premature ovarian insufficiency.[24] Primary amenorrhea or premature ovarian insufficiency prior to age 30 usually does not present in premutation carriers, and many of them will become pregnant and have children. The CGG repeats in premutation female carriers can expand to greater than 200 repeats during oogenesis, and increase the chance of conceiving a child with the fragile X syndrome (see Chapter 3). Because of the widespread implications of the fragile X premutation, as it affects both the woman and her offspring, and has implications for the rest of the family, all women who present with premature ovarian insufficiency should have their CGG repeat number determined. A woman found to be a premutation carrier should be counseled about its implications for her and for her offspring, and she should be encouraged to bring her family members for counseling and testing. Counseling of men who are premutation carriers is equally important.

Kelly was counseled that approximately 20% of women who are premutation carriers will develop premature ovarian insufficiency. Her elevated FSH and LH values are suspicious for diminished ovarian reserves. This may account for her difficulty in conceiving, although she still reports having periods, and pregnancies are known to occur to women with the diagnosis of premature ovarian insufficiency. If she conceives, there is a risk of premutation expanding to the full mutation and resulting in fragile X syndrome. The empiric risk of premutation expansion to the full mutation is approximately 5% with 64 CGG repeats.

Kelly also wanted to know her options for prenatal diagnosis if she conceives. Kelly can have CVS or amniocentesis to determine the CGG repeat status in the fetus, and to rule out expansion to the full mutation. Preimplantation genetic testing for fragile X syndrome is possible, but can be technically challenging due to allele dropout (one of the alleles may not amplify or be detectable) with expanding CGG repeats. Her family history is suspicious that maternal aunt with mild mental retardation may have a full mutation. Women with full mutations can be symptomatic and present with mild mental retardation. Her other aunt may be a premutation carrier whose son inherited a full mutation and was diagnosed with "autism." Kelly was encouraged to discuss fragile X with her family and to have her relatives visit a genetics professional for counseling and testing.

■ AUTOSOMAL CAUSES OF OVARIAN DYSFUNCTION

A number of autosomal genes have been implicated in ovarian function and failure. Because individually these genes account for a very small subset of affected individuals, screening for such mutations is currently not indicated for women with idiopathic infertility and/or ovarian failure. However, if family history and endocrine evaluations are consistent with mutations in a particular pathway, then a genetic work up should consider the genes discussed below to help determine a precise genetic pathology. We have divided genes important in fertility based on the phenotype of hypogonadotropic hypogonadism (low LH and FSH levels causing secondary ovarian dysfunction) and hypergonadotropic hypogonadism (elevated FSH and LH with primary pathology in the ovary).

Hypogonadotropic Hypogonadism

The hypothalamic-pituitary-gonadal (HPG) axis in females coordinates ovarian follicle maturation beyond the antral follicle with sexual behavior, and the physiologic preparation for pregnancy. Prior to a mature HPG axis, follicles are recruited to grow from primordial follicles, but cannot form antral follicles without sufficient gonadotropin stimulation. Spontaneous and targeted mutations in mice as well as genetic disorders in humans affecting hypothalamic and pituitary production of various peptides and hormones, have provided important insight into the hormonal regulation of folliculogenesis (Figure 14-1).

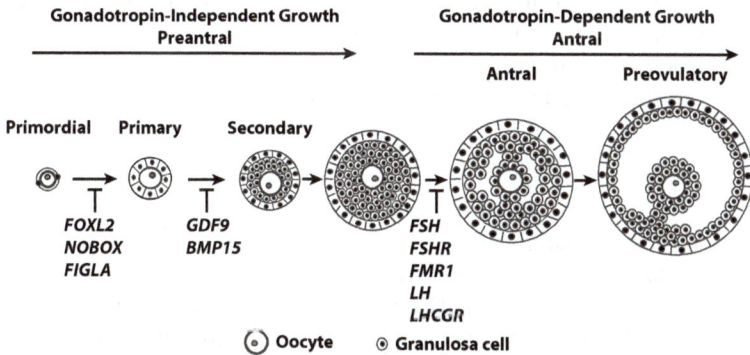

FIGURE 14-1. Ovarian folliculogenesis and genes implicated in ovarian failure. From left to right, follicle growth and activation begins when primordial follicles (small oocytes enveloped with flat granulosa cell layer) are recruited to form primary and subsequently larger follicles. Prior to antrum formation, follicle growth is independent of pituitary gonadotropins. Following ovulation, granulosa cells undergo luteinization to become the corpus luteum. A subset of genes implicated at various stages of follicular development has been associated with human ovarian failure and are listed at the point where ovarian folliculogenesis is thought to be disrupted. BMP-15, bone morphogenetic protein 15; FIGLA, factor in the germline alpha; FMR1, fragile X and mental retardation syndrome 1; FOXL2, forkhead box L2; FSH, follicle stimulating hormone; FSHR, follicle stimulating hormone receptor; GDF9, growth differentiation factor 9; LH, luteinizing hormone; LHCGR, luteinizing hormone/choriogonadotropin receptor; NOBOX, newborn ovary homeobox gene.

Gonadotropin Releasing Hormone

Gonadotropin releasing hormone (GnRH) is a decapeptide secreted by hypo-thalamic neurons in a pulsatile manner into the capillary plexus of the median eminence, and affects the release of LH and FSH from gonadotropic cells of the anterior pituitary. Humans with Kallmann syndrome, characterized by lack of GnRH, have hypogonadotropic (low levels of FSH and LH) hypogonadism.[26,27] Kallmann syndrome is a genetically heterogeneous disorder with X-linked, autosomal dominant, and autosomal recessive inheritance, and occurs as a result of defective migration in GnRH producing neurons and olfactory neurons.[26]

Gonadotropin Releasing Hormone Receptor

Gonadotropin releasing hormone receptor (GnRHR) mutations in humans cause infertility.[28] Several mutations have been described to date, and most are com-pound heterozygotes, with more severe phenotypes observed in homozygous mutations. Folliculogenesis is affected, but the degree of ovarian and follicle devel-opment is not clear due to difficulty in obtaining human ovaries for analysis. In one affected woman, small ovaries were detected with the presence of primordial follicles.

Follicle Stimulating Hormone

The pituitary glycoprotein follicle stimulating hormone (FSH) plays an essen-tial role in reproduction through interaction with gonadal FSH receptors. FSH is a dimeric glycoprotein composed of a unique beta subunit complexed with a common alpha subunit that is shared with thyroid stimulating hormone, lutein-izing hormone and chorionic gonadotropin. FSH binds to the FSH receptor and activates cell signals that lead to germ cell maturation and follicular growth.[29] Several women have been identified with mutations in FSH.[30,31] These women usually present with primary amenorrhea, absent breast development, low FSH, low estradiol, and high LH.

Luteinizing Hormone

Similar to FSH, luteinizing hormone (LH) is a glycoprotein hormone with a com-mon alpha subunit but a unique hormone-specific beta subunit and is synthe-sized in the pituitary gonadotropes. Mutations in LH beta subunit in humans are rare, and cause male hypogonadism and azoospermia, and female infertility.[32] The women with LH mutations that have been reported have normal pubertal development with secondary amenorrhea and infertility.[33]

Hypergonadotropic Hypogonadism

Follicle Stimulating Hormone receptor

Follicle stimulating hormone receptors (FSHRs) are transmembrane G (guanine nucleotide binding) protein coupled receptors. A Finish population-based study identified patients with autosomal recessive mutations in the FSHR gene as hav-ing XX gonadal dysgenesis (46,XX women with primary or secondary amenor-rhea and serum FSH >40 mIU/mL).[34] The overall frequency of the disorder in Finland was 1 per 8300 live born females, a relatively high incidence attributed to the **founder effect**, and FSHR mutation screening is clinically offered to Finnish women with hypergonadotropic hypogonadism. The **founder effect** occurs when a new population is established from a small number of individuals. FSHR mutations are rare in American women, and unless an individual is of Finnish origin, screening for FSHR mutations is not indicated at this time.

Luteinizing Hormone Receptor

Like FSH receptors, LH receptors are single chain transmembrane glycoproteins that belong to the G protein–coupled receptor family. Women with inactivating luteinizing hormone receptor (LHCGR) mutations have normal external genitalia, spontaneous breast and pubic hair development at puberty, and normal or late menarche followed by oligomenorrhea and infertility.[35,36] Estradiol and progesterone levels are normal for the early to midfollicular phase, but do not reach ovulatory or luteal phase levels. Serum LH levels are high, whereas follicle-stimulating hormone levels are normal or only slightly increased. Pelvic ultrasound usually demonstrates a small or normal uterus, and normal or enlarged ovaries with cysts.

■ SYNDROMIC CAUSES OF OVARIAN FAILURE

When ovarian failure is associated with extra gonadal manifestations and dysmorphic features, a possibility exists that infertility and ovarian failure are part of a syndrome. There are several well-known syndromes that associate with ovarian failure and infertility and the genes are listed in Table 14-1.

■ A PRACTICAL CLINICAL APPROACH TO INFERTILITY EVALUATIONS

Identification of genetic causes underlying male and female infertility is an essential part of the clinical evaluation, genetic counseling, and successful treatment of the infertile couple. Accurate genetic diagnosis presents an opportunity to guide treatment options, to achieve natural conception with their own gametes, and to provide important information regarding the health and

■ TABLE 14-1. Genetic Syndromes that Cause Premature Ovarian Failure

Syndrome	Gene
Fanconi Anemia	FANCA
Ataxia-telangiectasia	ATM
Bloom syndrome	BLM
Aromatase deficiency	CYP19A1
Werner syndrome	WRN
Martsolf syndrome	RAB3GAP2
Galactosemia	GALT
BPES, Type I	FOXL2

reproductive potential of an affected individual. Moreover, genetic counseling of the couple is essential to discuss the risk of transmitting a genetic abnormality to the offspring. A genetic evaluation is indicated for couples that fail to achieve pregnancy after 12 months of regular unprotected intercourse, as well as for patients with a clinical diagnosis or medical history of a chromosomal or genetic disorder. A careful family history is necessary to determine if there is a clear familial pattern of infertility, miscarriages, skewed gender ratios (eg, complete androgen insensitivity syndrome), accelerated aging, or syndromic causes associated with infertility (Fanconi anemia, Bloom syndrome, ataxia telangiectasia). However, a negative family history does not rule out a genetic contribution, as *de novo* genetic events likely account for a substantial number of sporadic cases. Examples include most chromosomal abnormalities, such as Klinefelter syndrome. A karyotype analysis should be performed as an initial component of evaluation for male or female infertility to identify sex chromosome aneuploidy and gross structural chromosome rearrangements. Despite gonadal failure in most affected patients with Klinefelter and Turner syndrome, 5% to 20% of individuals with sex chromosome aneuploidy may have limited number of mature germ cells, enabling live birth of biological children. The number of available germ cells significantly decreases with age. Cryopreservation of ovarian follicles or retrieved testicular spermatozoa as an infertility treatment option may be feasible for some patients with Turner or Klinefelter syndrome, respectively.

Structural chromosome abnormalities detected by karyotype analysis confer an increased risk for spermatogenic failure, miscarriages, stillbirth, and live born children with congenital defects and chromosomal aberrations. In some patients, balanced chromosome abnormalities are present; however, they are below the resolution of detection by conventional cytogenetic analysis. Microarray analysis should be considered on DNA from spontaneous abortions and stillbirths, if available. FISH analysis on sperm cells from a male carrier of a structural chromosome rearrangement will help determine chromosome segregation patterns, the likelihood of abnormal chromosome complement in the embryo, and determine the best approach to preimplantation genetic diagnosis (PGD).

In the case of a normal karyotype, expanded genetic testing should include microarray analysis to detect submicroscopic chromosome abnormalities, and depending on the clinical information, a possible individual gene mutation analysis. It is critical that men with nonobstructive azoospermia or oligospermia undergo molecular and cytogenetics analyses for Y chromosome rearrangements and microdeletions in order to receive accurate diagnosis and proper genetic counseling prior to assisted reproduction.

High-resolution whole genome microarray analyses are recommended as a part of genetic evaluation of infertility in patients with normal karyotype. *FMR1* testing for the fragile X to rule out premutation carrier status is recommended for all women with cessation of menses and elevated gonadotropin levels prior to age 40. It is important to note that negative genetic testing does not exclude genetic pathology, as there are other, presently unknown, genes that are implicated in normal gametogenesis. To date, mutations in approximately 300 genes are known to associate with reproductive disorders, and this list will continue to grow.

Genetic counseling should be ideally provided before the genetic test is offered, so that the couple understands the *benefits and limitations* of genetic testing. Post-test genetic counseling is necessary for the couple to understand the significance of each possible outcome: normal results, pathologic test findings, and findings of unknown clinical significance. It is essential that gynecologists are engaged with clinical genetics experts, including genomic laboratories, in order to provide the most optimal and appropriate testing to their patients.

> **Case 4: Ms. Roberts is a 37-year-old G_4P_{2022} who recently miscarried at 10 weeks' gestation. She had two full-term pregnancies, 10 and 12 years ago. She divorced the father of these children, and 2 years ago she remarried and has been attempting to have a child with her new spouse. Six months ago, she had a spontaneous loss at 6 weeks' gestation, and no pathologic evaluation was done on the products of conception. Her second loss was sent for chromosome studies, and indicated trisomy 22. Her family history is negative for any history of recurrent pregnancy loss, birth defects, or apparent inherited conditions. She has no history of medical illnesses, or surgeries, and takes no medications. She is concerned about the two miscarriages, and wants to know if she and her husband should have genetic studies.**

Spontaneous abortion is defined as pregnancy loss prior to 20 weeks' gestation, and occurs in 15% to 25% of clinically recognized pregnancies. Of those losses occurring in the first trimester, the great majority are random chromosome errors, most being trisomies, monosomies, and polyploidy. Because of this high rate of natural losses from random genetic events, it is not uncommon for a patient to have more than one miscarriage in her reproductive career. Many different definitions have been put forward as to what constitutes "recurrent pregnancy loss," but these authors use a more liberal definition of two or more failed clinical pregnancies to determine who needs a "genetic" evaluation, as will be outlined below.

Genetic Causes of Pregnancy Loss

Cytogenetic abnormalities are the most common cause of pregnancy loss with approximately 60% of early losses having a numerical chromosome abnormality. In patients above the age of 35, 75% to 80% of first-trimester losses will be cytogenetically abnormal. On the other hand, unbalanced structural chromosomal abnormalities are found in less than 10% of products of conception, and less than half of these result from a parent with a balanced translocation or other structural abnormality. Therefore, blood chromosomes on a couple with recurrent pregnancy loss will have a yield in the range of 2% to 5%.[37]

Chromosome analysis of products of conception (POC) can be an excellent diagnostic tool in some institutions, but have a dismal yield in others. Two factors appear to explain most of the discrepancy. Laboratories that have experience with chorionic villus samples, and evaluate POC in the same fashion, will dissect away decidua and culture only fetal or placental material. A normal female karyotype in these laboratories more likely reflects the POC result, and not maternal chromosome results. Even in experienced laboratories, viability of the tissue is a significant problem, and culture failure will occur relatively frequently. Therefore, most laboratories are shifting away from traditional cytogenetic methods toward molecular techniques, such as microarray, which do not require culturing of the POC.

Our approach to the patient with "recurrent loss" is to test the POC of the second and subsequent losses. The finding of a sporadic chromosome abnormality provides an explanation of the loss, and therefore no further evaluation is necessary. In younger patients with recurrent aneuploidy, there are at least three explanations. First, the losses are all random, and the couple is simply "unlucky." Second, if the same aneuploidy, such as trisomy 21, is seen in each loss, then one member of the couple may have either somatic or germ cell mosaicism. Blood chromosomes on the couple may detect the presence of somatic mosaicism in one of them, but there are currently no techniques to accurately detect germ cell mosaicism. The third possibility for recurrent aneuploidy involving more than one chromosome is that one member of the couple carries a gene mutation that causes recurrent meiotic failure. Currently there are no diagnostic tests to assess for this possibility.

To date there are no specific gene mutations that are known to directly cause recurrent pregnancy loss only. However, there are a number of X-linked conditions that are inherited in an X-linked dominant fashion. In these conditions, the mutation is manifest in females, but in males is lethal (eg, incontinentia pigmenti due to mutations in the X-linked IKBKG gene). Some of these conditions may progress far enough in pregnancy to be detected by ultrasound (X-linked multiple pterygium syndrome), but most end in early embryo death. A family history of multiple females with early pregnancy loss, and evidence of skewed gender ratio (limited male offspring) should prompt a referral to a geneticist for further evaluation.

As we have noted in several locations in this book, this area is one where genome-wide sequencing is likely to yield many gene mutations that are lethal, and most will likely be recessive (requiring two copies of the mutated gene). The practicing physician should seek consultation from specialists in pregnancy loss whenever the history is suggestive of a genetic cause of the losses.

In counseling Ms. Roberts it is important to reassure her that the recent loss was a sporadic event, and not related to heritable genetic condition. Likewise, she can be counseled that given her age, the first loss was likely also due to chromosomal aneuploidy. Although her risk for another aneuploid pregnancy is no greater than anyone else of similar age, it must be emphasized that risk of miscarriage does increase with age due to the increase risk of nondisjunction and other nongenetic factors. In women above 40, the rate of miscarriage approaches 50%.[38]

REFERENCES

1. Turek PJ. Practical approaches to the diagnosis and management of male infertility. *Nat Clin Pract Urol*. 2005;2:226-238.

2. de Kretser DM. Male infertility. *Lancet*. 1997;349:787-790.

3. Anderson JE, Farr SL, Jamieson DJ, et al. Infertility services reported by men in the United States: national survey data. *Fertil Steril*. 2009;91:2466-2470.

4. McLachlan RI , O'Bryan MK. State of the art for genetic testing of infertile men. *J Clin Endocrinol Metab*. 2010;95:1013-1024.

5. Harton GL, Tempest HG. Chromosomal disorders and male infertility. *Asian J Androl*. 2012;14:32-39.

6. Walsh TJ, Pera RR, Turek PJ. The genetics of male infertility. *Semin Reprod Med*. 2009;27:124-136.

7. Wikstrom AM, Dunkel L. Testicular function in Klinefelter syndrome. *Horm Res*. 2008;69:317-326.

8. O'Flynn O'Brien KL, Varghese AC, Agarwal A. The genetic causes of male factor infertility: a review. *Fertil Steril*. 2010;93:1-12.

9. Martin RH. Cytogenetic determinants of male fertility. *Hum Reprod Update*. 2008;14:379-390.

10. Hennebicq S, Pelletier R, Bergues U, et al. Risk of trisomy 21 in offspring of patients with Klinefelter's syndrome. *Lancet*. 2001;357:2104-2105.

11. Kuroda-Kawaguchi T, Skaletsky H, Brown LG, et al. The AZFc region of the Y chromosome features massive palindromes and uniform recurrent deletions in infertile men. *Nat Genet*. 2001;29:279-286.

12. Hann MC, Lau PE, Tempest HG. Meiotic recombination and male infertility: from basic science to clinical reality? *Asian J Androl*. 2011;13:212-218.

13. Marchetti F, Wyrobek AJ. Mechanisms and consequences of paternally-transmitted chromosomal abnormalities. *Birth Defects Res C Embryo Today*. 2005;75: 112-129.

14. Madan K. Balanced complex chromosome rearrangements: reproductive aspects. A review. *Am J Med Genet Part A*. 2012;158A:947-963.

15. Roux C, Tripogney C, Morel F, et al. Segregation of chromosomes in sperm of Robertsonian translocation carriers. *Cytogenet Genome Res*. 2005;111:291-296.

16. Engels H, Eggermann T, Caliebe A, et al. Genetic counseling in Robertsonian translocations der(13;14): frequencies of reproductive outcomes and infertility in 101 pedigrees. *Am J Med Genet Part A*. 2008;146A:2611-2616.

17. Simpson JL, Rajkovic A. Ovarian differentiation and gonadal failure. *Am J Med Genet*. 1999;89:186-200.

18. Nelson LM. Clinical practice. Primary ovarian insufficiency. *N Engl J Med*. 2009;360:606-614.

19. van der Schouw YT, van der Graaf Y, Steyerberg EW, et al. Age at menopause as a risk factor for cardiovascular mortality. *Lancet*. 1996;347:714-718.

20. Anasti JN, Kalantaridou SN, Kimzey LM, et al. L.M. Bone loss in young women with karyotypically normal spontaneous premature ovarian failure. *Obstet Gynecol*. 1998;91:12-15.

21. Uygur D, Sengul O, Bayar D, et al. Bone loss in young women with premature ovarian failure. *Arch Gynecol Obstet*. 2005;273:17-19.

22. Jacobsen BK, Heuch I, Kvale G. Age at natural menopause and all-cause mortality: a 37-year follow-up of 19,731 Norwegian women. *Am J Epidemiol*. 2003;157: 923-929.

23. Heard E, Turner J. Function of the sex chromosomes in mammalian fertility. *Cold Spring Harb Perspect Biol*. 2011 Oct 1;3(10):a002675.

24. Toniolo D, Rizzolio F. X chromosome and ovarian failure. *Semin Reprod Med*. 2007;25:264-271.

25. Tartaglia NR, Howell S, Sutherland A, et al. A review of trisomy X (47,XXX). *Orphanet J Rare Dis*. 2010;5:8.

26. McKusick VA. 308700 Kallmann syndrome. In: McKusick VA. *Mendelian Inheritance in Man*. Baltimore, MD: Johns Hopkins University Press; 1994.

27. Persson JW, Humphrey K, Watson C, et al. Investigation of a unique male and female sibship with Kallmann's syndrome and 46,XX gonadal dysgenesis with short stature. *Hum Reprod*. 1999;14:1207-1212.

28. de Roux N, Milgrom E. Inherited disorders of GnRH and gonadotropin receptors. *Mol Cell Endocrinol*. 2001;179:83-87.

29. Findlay JK, Drummond AE. Regulation of the FSH receptor in the ovary. *Trends Endocrinol Met*. 1999;10:183-188.

30. Matthews CH, Borgato S, Beck-Peccoz P, et al. Primary amenorrhoea and infertility due to a mutation in the beta- subunit of follicle-stimulating hormone. *Nat Genet*. 1993;5:83-86.

31. Layman LC, Lee EJ, Peak DB, et al. Delayed puberty and hypogonadism caused by mutations in the follicle-stimulating hormone beta-subunit gene. *N Engl J Med*. 1997;337:607-611.

32. Weiss J, Axelrod L, Whitcomb RW, et al. Hypogonadism caused by a single amino acid substitution in the beta subunit of luteinizing hormone. *N Engl J Med*. 1992;326:179-183.

33. Lofrano-Porto A, Barra GB, Giacomini LA, et al. Luteinizing hormone beta mutation and hypogonadism in men and women. *N Engl J Med*. 2007;357:897-904.

34. Aittomaki K, Lucena JL, Pakarinen P, et al. Mutation in the follicle-stimulating hormone receptor gene causes hereditary hypergonadotropic ovarian failure. *Cell*. 1995;82:959-968.

35. Latronico AC, Anasti J, Arnhold IJ, et al. Brief report: testicular and ovarian resistance to luteinizing hormone caused by inactivating mutations of the luteinizing hormone-receptor gene. *N Engl J Med*. 1996;334:507-512.

36. Toledo SP, Brunner HG, Kraaij R, et al. An inactivating mutation of the luteinizing hormone receptor causes amenorrhea in a 46,XX female. *J Clin Endocrinol Metab*. 1996;81:3850-3854.

37. The Practice Committee of the American Society for Reproductive Medicine. Evaluation and treatment of recurrent pregnancy loss: a committee opinion. *Fertil Steril*. 2012;98:1103-1111.

38. Nybo Andersen AM, Wohlfahrt J, Christens P, et al: Maternal age and fetal loss: population based register linkage study. *BMJ*. 2000;320:1708-1712.

Methods of
Genetic Testing

CHAPTER

15

Methods of
Modern Cytogenetics

- ■ G-BANDED KARYOTYPE ANALYSIS
- ■ CHROMOSOMAL MICROARRAY ANALYSIS
- ■ FLUORESCENCE IN SITU HYBRIDIZATION (FISH) ANALYSIS
- ■ APPLICATIONS

Prenatal and Postnatal Diagnosis
Miscarriage and Stillbirth

Case 1: Ms. Sanfilippo is a 25-year-old gravida 5 para 3104 whose first-trimester screen gave her a 1:1200 risk of Down syndrome and <1:5000 risk of trisomy 18, and a second-trimester alpha fetoprotein was in the normal range (1.2 MOM). She has no significant past medical history. Her obstetric history was significant for a previous term spontaneous vaginal delivery complicated by a rectovaginal fistula. This was followed by a term cesarean delivery, and her last pregnancy was a preterm repeat cesarean at 34 weeks. A three generation family history was significant for Hirschsprung disease in a son with a previous partner. An initial anatomy ultrasound at 18 weeks of gestation was performed at an outside hospital, and showed the fetus to have a left sided diaphragmatic hernia with cardiac displacement to the right side of the chest. The patient was referred to a regional center because of the abnormal ultrasound. A repeat ultrasound at 20 weeks of gestation identified a thickened nuchal fold of 7 mm, bilateral echogenic kidneys with nephromegaly, and a left-sided diaphragmatic hernia. Ms. Sanfilippo was counseled about the risks and benefits of amniocentesis. Rapid FISH analysis was performed on 50 interphase cells from the amniotic fluid with #13, #18, #21, X-, and Y-specific probes. No evidence of trisomy 13, 18, or 21 was detected. Analysis of the X and Y probe revealed two copies of the X probe and no copies of the Y probe, consistent with 46,XX female karyotype. FISH analysis was also performed using probes specific for chromosome 12 to rule out mosaic isochromosome 12p (Pallister-Killian syndrome), and the results were consistent with normal chromosome 12. Fifteen cells were analyzed from the amniotic fluid specimen. No significant numerical or structural aberrations were seen at the 475 G-band level of resolution. The karyotype was reported as normal, 46,XX female. Since the karyotype and FISH results were both normal, an oligonucleotide microarray was performed. Microarray-based comparative genomic hybridization (aCGH), also known as chromosomal microarray technique (CMA) was performed using a 135K-feature whole-genome microarray. Microarray revealed a 1.4-Mb deletion on 17q12. Neither parent carried the deletion; therefore this deletion was a de novo finding. The deletion caused haploinsufficiency for 17 genes, including *AATF, ACACA, DDX52, DUSP14, GGNBP2, HNF1B, LHX1, PIGW, SYNRG, TADA2A,* and *ZNHIT3*. The deleted region on 17q12 is similar in size and gene content to the previously reported 17q12 microdeletion syndrome.[1] The 17q12 microdeletion syndrome has been associated with MODY5 (maturity-onset of diabetes of the young, type 5), cystic renal disease, pancreatic atrophy, liver abnormalities, cognitive impairment, and structural brain abnormalities. Ms. Sanfilippo was counseled with regards to the diagnosis and prognosis. The risk of recurrence is at most 2% to 3%, as gonadal mosaicism cannot be ruled out. After reviewing the risks and prognosis associated with congenital diaphragmatic hernia and 17q12 microdeletion syndrome, Ms. Sanfilippo opted for comfort measures after her baby is born.

Chromosomal abnormalities occur in germ cell division (meiosis), during early fetal development, or after birth in any cell in the body (mitosis) (see Chapter 2). The number, structure, properties of chromosomes, chromosomal behavior, and influence of chromosomal abnormalities on the phenotype are studied in cytogenetics. The analysis of chromosomes in human development and disease is accomplished through classical cytogenetic procedures, including Giemsa or G-banding karyotype analysis and C-(constitutive heterochromatin) banding. Molecular techniques such as array comparative genomic hybridization (aCGH/ CMA) and single nucleotide polymorphism microarray (SNP microarray) analyses have improved resolution, and have replaced the karyotype in many clinical situations as the first line technique to detect genomic imbalances.

■ G-BANDED KARYOTYPE ANALYSIS

Cells duplicate their genetic material and generate genetically identical daughter cells during mitosis. Chromosome morphology can be visualized and studied under the light microscope during the prophase or metaphase of the mitotic cell division, when chromosomes are condensed. During metaphase, replicated chromosomes are aligned and sister chromatids are ready for separation to the opposite poles along the spindle fibers. Colchicine, a spindle inhibitor, added to the cell culture, disrupts the spindle-fiber complex and arrests mitosis. The

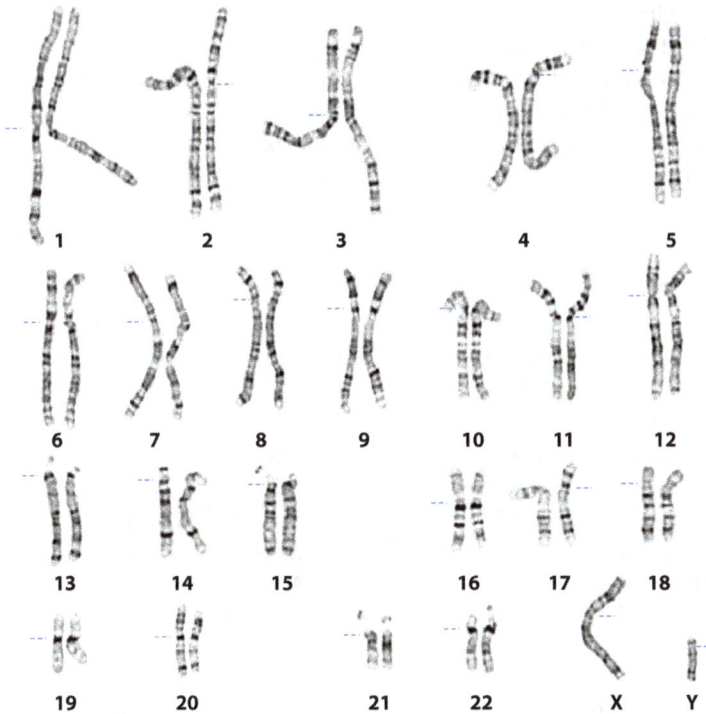

FIGURE 15-1. A human normal male karyotype. Homologous chromosomes (homo-logues), the two chromosomes in a pair of autosomes, are composed of similar (but not identical) DNA sequences. Each homologue encodes the same set of genes in the same order, but may contain different variant forms of the same gene (allele), as well as variable noncoding DNA (introns). Centromeres are indicated by the dashed lines, separating the short and long arms.

chromosomes, when stained with a dye (Giemsa), have a distinct banded pattern (G-banding) that provides a unique bar code to each chromosome (Figure 15-1). Chromosomes become gradually shortened as the cell cycle progresses from inter-phase to metaphase. Depending on the degree of chromosome condensation, the chromosomes reveal from 400 to 850 bands per haploid genome, which enables detection of chromosomal alterations with resolution to the 5 to 10 Mb level by routine microscopic analysis. High-resolution chromosome studies (600-850 bands) allow a more detailed analysis of the chromosome structure, as compared to the 400 to 550 bands observed with routine metaphase banding. The karyotype provides an overview of the whole genome and detects both numerical and gross structural chromosomal aberrations.

Karyotyping requires viable tissue samples to establish cell culture, and induce mitosis, followed by cell harvesting, chromosome banding, and microscopic analysis. White blood cells, particularly T-lymphocytes, stimulated by phytohemagglu-tinin (PHA), rapidly divide during 48 to 72 hours of incubation and produce good quality high-resolution metaphases. In short-term blood cultures, mitogen-stimulated cells divide from one to five times, while tissues derived from chorionic villi, amniocytes, and fibroblasts undergo 20 to 100 mitotic cell divisions. Because of numerous cell divisions, some cells may undergo abnormal division and introduce a cell line with abnormal chromosome structure or number. These *in vitro* cultural artifacts lead to pseudomosaicism (see Chapter 2). Minimizing the time of a sample in culture provides cytogenetic results that most closely reflect *in vivo* conditions.

■ CHROMOSOMAL MICROARRAY ANALYSIS

Chromosomal microarray analysis (CMA), also known as array-based comparative genomic hybridization (aCGH), is a technique to detect DNA copy number variations (CNVs) in the whole genome at a high resolution. In CMA, genomic DNA of the test sample is labeled with one fluorescent dye and control (reference) diploid DNA is labeled with another fluorescent dye (Figure 15-2). Equal amounts of the test and control DNA are cohybridized to a set of genomic fragments (oligonucleotide probes) spotted on a glass slide (array). The intensities of fluorescent dyes at each probe are measured by a scanner and compared between the test DNA and control DNA. If the intensities are equal at the given probe, the amount of the test DNA is interpreted as normal. Increased or decreased intensity for the test DNA over a control DNA indicates gain or loss in DNA amount respectively (Figure 15-2D, E). Most current CMA platforms contain from 60,000 to 400,000 oligonucleotide probes with comprehensive probe coverage within clinically relevant genes, as well as limited probes for the rest of the genome. CMA reliably detects DNA losses (deletions) and gains (duplications and triplications) as small as 200 kb in size, which gives at least 25-fold better resolution than G-banded chromosome analysis. The resolution of CMA depends on the total number of probes and average probe spacing across the genome. CMA can detect aneuploidy (monosomy and trisomy) and unbalanced structural rearrangements such as deletions, duplications, triplications, unbalanced insertions, isochromosomes, marker chromosomes, and complex chromosome abnormalities, but cannot detect balanced rearrangements or polyploidy. Arrays based on single nucleotide polymorphisms (SNP arrays), and the combination of oligonucleotide and SNP arrays, can detect the same abnormalities as CMA, as well as triploidies and copy number neutral chromosome abnormalities, such as contiguous regions of homozygosity that occur with uniparental isodisomy (UPD), consanguinity, or complete molar pregnancy. CMA, unlike G-banded karyotype, does not require cell culture, and can be completed within 3 to 5 days.

It is important to remember that CMA will not detect balanced rearrangements such as balanced translocations, balanced inversions and balanced insertions, because the technique does not allow visualization of chromosomal structure, but only provides information on genomic content.[2] An additional limitation of CMA is the detection of mosaicism. Mosaicism less than 10% is likely to be missed by CMA.[3,4]

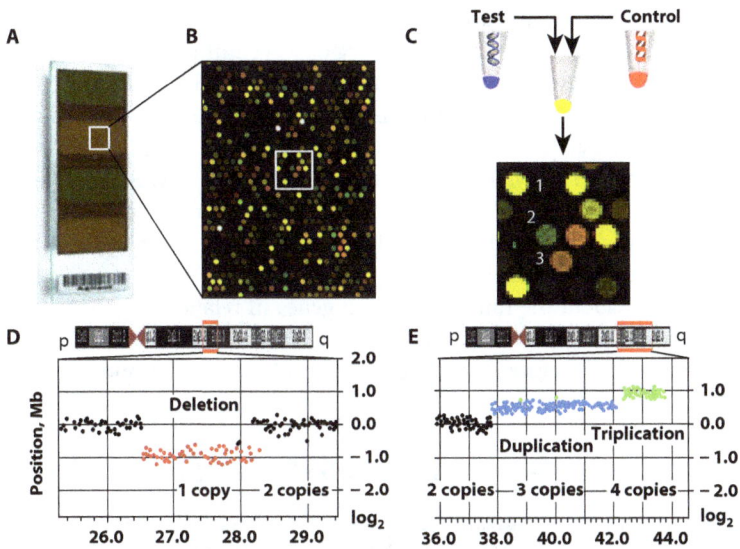

FIGURE 15-2. **The array comparative genomic hybridization (aCGH/CMA) technology.** **(A)** A DNA microarray is usually a microscope slide with a set of short DNA fragments from selected regions of the genome spotted onto a surface. **(B)** A magnified view of the micro-array surface after hybridization. **(C)** Genomic DNAs from the test (patient) and a control (normal individual of the same gender) samples are differentially labeled using Cy3 and Cy5 dyes, mixed, and hybridized into array. Spots with an equal amount of Cy3 and Cy5 (spot 1) appear yellow, while spots with an extra amount of test DNA look green (spot 2), and spots where amount of a test DNA is decreased appear red (spot 3). **(D)** Array CGH plot showing a deletion. Probes (black and red dots) are aligned along the X axis according to the physical position on the chromosome (from the short to the long arm). Ratio between the intensity of Cy3 and Cy5 for each probe is calculated and values are placed onto a $\log_2$ scale (Y axis). Probes with an equal amount of the test and control DNA (black dots, ratio = 2/2, $\log_2(2/2) = 0$) are clustered around a "0" score on the $\log_2$ scale. Negative $\log_2$ score indicates deletion (red dots, ratio = 1/2, $\log_2(1/2) = -1.0$). **(E)** Array CGH plot showing a complex duplication/ triplication rearrangement. Gain in DNA copy number is seen as positive $\log_2$ scores. Blue dots represent duplication (ratio = 3/2, $\log_2(3/2) = 0.58$). Green dots (ratio = 4/2, $\log_2(4/2) = 1.0$) depict a triplication (total 4 copies of DNA).

CMA technology has enabled discovery of more than 300 microdeletion and microduplication syndromes.[4] Benign copy-number variants (CNVs) ranging from 1 kb to ~1 Mb in size are also abundantly present in genomes of healthy individuals. Benign CNVs are usually inherited and encompass as much as 12% of the genome. In the course of interpreting CMA findings, it is useful to divide DNA copy number variations as **pathogenic**, **benign**, or of **unclear clinical significance**. Pathogenic CNVs are derived from known, dosage sensitive genes, associated with abnormal phenotypes, such as, for example, microdeletions of the 7q11.23, 9q34, 22q11.21 regions and microduplications of 17p12 and Xq28, resulting in Williams-Beuren (OMIM 194050), Kleefstra (OMIM 610253), DiGeorge (OMIM 188400), Charcot-Marie-Tooth disease, type 1A (OMIM

118220), and Lubs X-linked mental retardation (OMIM 300260) syndromes, respectively. Benign CNVs are commonly observed in populations of healthy individuals and have been catalogued in publicly available databases. CMA also may detect rare or novel CNVs for which there is no clinical information and they are classified as CNVs of uncertain clinical significance. If such a CNV is inherited from a phenotypically normal parent, the CNV is less likely to cause pathology. However, if such a CNV is not found in parents, but found in the affected child (*de novo*), and associated with developmental or structural physical abnormality, careful analysis of the genes that are deleted or duplicated and what is known about the function of such genes in relationship to the affected phenotype, may help in the interpretation of causality. Interpretation of rare/novel CNVs often requires genetic evaluation of the parents and other family members.[5]

■ FLUORESCENCE IN SITU HYBRIDIZATION (FISH) ANALYSIS

Fluorescence *in situ* hybridization is a molecular cytogenetic technique in which DNA fragments of 40 to 250 kb are labeled with fluorescent dye and used to interrogate genomic imbalances in a specific chromosomal region. Fluorescent signals are visualized and studied using a fluorescent microscope (Figure 15-3). FISH analysis can be performed on metaphase chromosomes, interphase nuclei, or extended chromatin fibers, and has been a useful adjunct tool to a classic karyotype to determine submicroscopic deletions/duplications in known disease loci.

FISH analysis is currently performed when a specific syndrome is suspected based on clinical presentation or a positive family history of a microdeletion that can be diagnosed with specific FISH probes. Moreover, FISH technique can be used for rapid detection of common trisomies for chromosomes 13, 18, 21, and sex chromosome aneuploidies. Using probes specific for these chromosomes (locus and centromere specific), FISH analysis can be performed on uncultured (interphase) cells from amniotic fluid or CVS samples to obtain results within a 48-hour period (Figure 15-3D). In rare instances, FISH may provide false negative results when structurally abnormal chromosomes are present, and chromosomal array or classic karyotype should follow a negative FISH analysis. FISH analysis also can be performed on a paraffin-embedded tissue, particularly from products of conceptions, to establish ploidy of the fetus (Figure 15-3) or on tumor cells. Another advantage of the FISH technique is ability to study individual cells and identify low-level mosaicism for an abnormal cell population.

FISH can be used to screen embryos for common sporadic chromosome aneuploidy, or to detect a specific chromosomal abnormality, known as preimplantation genetic screening (PGS) or preimplantation genetic diagnosis (PGD), respectively. In assisted reproduction, genetically balanced embryos can be selected to achieve successful pregnancy from parent who carries a chromosomal abnormality.

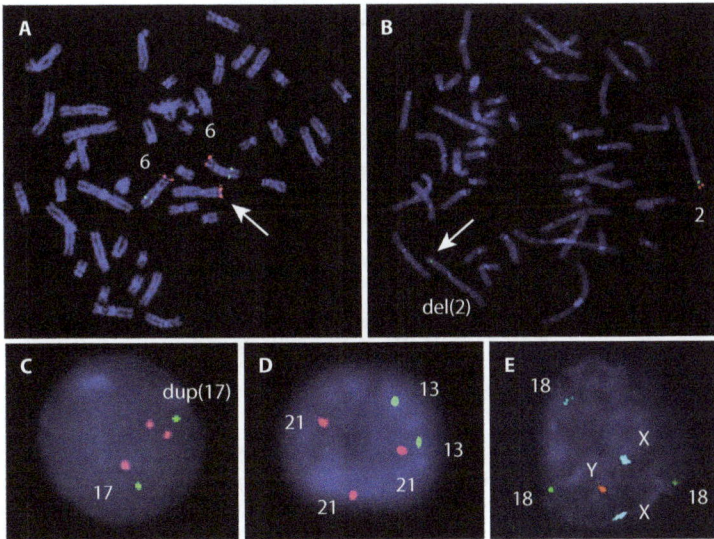

FIGURE 15-3. Chromosome aberrations detected by FISH analysis. (A) Two-color metaphase analysis reveals an unbalanced chromosome rearrangement in a patient with normal karyotype. FISH analysis using probes mapped to the terminal 6p region (red) and a control probe, located at the long arm of chromosome 6 (green), detected an additional red signal on the short arm of chromosome 2 (arrow). **(B)** FISH analysis with the chromosome 2 locus-specific probes showing the red and green signals on the normal chromosome 2. Red signal is absent on the second chromosome 2 (arrow) indicating a deletion on the terminal short arm. **(C)** A duplication involving the 17p11.2 region (red signal) is detected on interphase cells from a patient with Charcot-Marie-Tooth 1A disease. **(D)** FISH analysis of interphase amniotic fluid cells detecting three signals for chromosome 21 (red) and two signals for 13 (green), indicating a fetus with trisomy 21. **(E)** Multicolor FISH analysis on paraffin-embedded tissue sections from a missed abortion showing three copies of chromosome 18 (blue signal) and a total three sex chromosomes: two copies of the X chromosome (green signal) and one copy of the Y chromosome (red), indicating a fetus with triploidy.

■ APPLICATIONS

Prenatal and Postnatal Diagnosis

In prenatal diagnosis, chorionic villi and amniotic fluid, and rarely fetal blood derived from percutaneous umbilical blood sampling, are used to detect chromosome abnormalities in a fetus. Among women referred for cytogenetic testing due to advanced maternal age, abnormal maternal serum screening, or fetal anomalies detected by ultrasound, approximately 1 in 10 of fetuses are found to have chromosome abnormalities. CMA has a higher diagnostic yield than conventional karyotype.[5,6] In the presence of a structural fetal anomaly and normal G-banded karyotype, CMA reveals clinically relevant deletions or duplications in 6.0% of fetal samples. Moreover, in individuals who had normal karyotype on amniocentesis samples obtained for the indications of advanced maternal age or positive first- or second-trimester screening results, the CMA yields clinically significant

Prenatal diagnostic testing guidelines flow chart

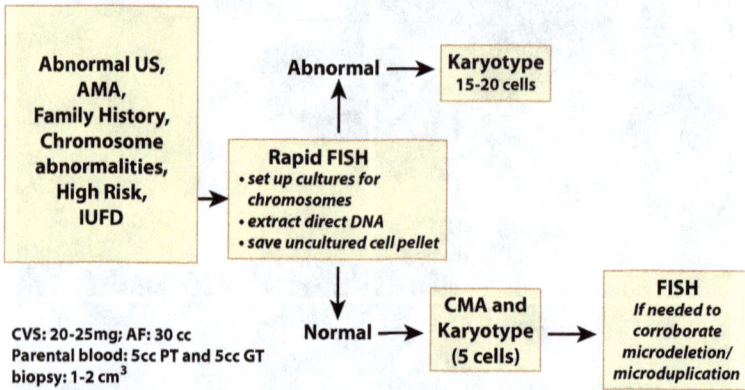

FIGURE 15-4. Prenatal testing guideline flow chart. Individuals present to the clinic for diagnostic prenatal testing due to various indications. Rapid FISH technique can be used for rapid detection of common trisomies for chromosomes 13, 18, 21, and sex chromosome aneuploidies (48 hours). If rapid FISH uncovers an aneuploidy, full karyotyping will be done to corroborate the findings and determine if the aneuploidy is due to a translocation. If rapid FISH results are interpreted as normal, chromosomal microarray (CMA) can be ordered to determine if genomic imbalances (microdeletions/microduplications) are present in the fetal genome. Limited karyotype analysis on five cells can help determine the overall chromosome architecture, and presence of structural aberrations. FISH analysis is currently used to corroborate CMA findings.

findings in almost 2% of cases.[6] CMA is recommended as a first tier diagnostic test in individuals with postnatal diagnosis of congenital anomalies, developmental delay or intellectual disabilities, and autism spectrum disorders.[4] Moreover, CMA is an appropriate first tier test in prenatal diagnosis of structural fetal anomalies detected by ultrasound. A flow chart (Figure 15-4) shows a reasonable strategy in a patient who carries a fetus with structural anomalies. Rapid FISH on amniotic fluid or chorionic villi will rule out aneuploidy involving chromosomes 13, 18, 21, X, and Y in 48 hours, and can be followed by CMA to rule out microdeletions/microduplications, if rapid FISH is normal. A limited karyotype on five cells can also be done to rule out structural balanced rearrangements.

Miscarriage and Stillbirth

Chromosome studies of products of conception are essential to determine the cause of pregnancy loss and provide useful information about the recurrence risk for subsequent pregnancies. Chromosome abnormalities in spontaneous abortions occur in at least 50% to 60% of cases.[7,8] Autosomal trisomy, triploidy, and monosomy X account for most of the abnormalities with approximately 5% due to microscopically visible structural chromosome rearrangements. Karyotypic abnormalities in stillbirths, which are defined as a fetal death after 20 weeks of gestation, are identified in 6% to 13% of cases with a successful analysis. In stillbirths without obvious anomalies, the diagnostic yield is 6.5% and with anomalies it is close to 20%. Chromosomal microarrays raise the diagnostic yield to 8.8% without anomalies and 30% with anomalies. Chromosomal microarrays can be performed on nonviable tissues, which is a major advantage over classical chromosome analysis that requires viable tissues.

REFERENCES

1. Mefford HC, Clauin S, Sharp AJ, et al. Recurrent reciprocal genomic rearrangements of 17q12 are associated with renal disease, diabetes, and epilepsy. *Am J Hum Genet.* 2007;81:1057-1069.

2. Van den Veyver IB, Beaudet AL. Comparative genomic hybridization and prenatal diagnosis. *Curr Opin Obstet Gynecol.* 2006;18:185-191.

3. Stankiewicz P, Beaudet AL. Use of array CGH in the evaluation of dysmorphology, malformations, developmental delay, and idiopathic mental retardation. *Curr Opin Genet Dev.* 2007;17:182-192.

4. Miller DT, Adam MP, Aradhya S, et al. Consensus statement: chromosomal microarray is a first-tier clinical diagnostic test for individuals with developmental disabilities or congenital anomalies. *Am J Hum Genet.* 2010;86:749-764.

5. Yatsenko S, Davis S, Hendrix N, et al. Application of chromosomal microarray in the evaluation of abnormal prenatal findings. *Clin Genet.* 2013;84:47-54.

6. Wapner RJ, Martin CL, Levy B, et al. Chromosomal microarray versus karyotyping for prenatal diagnosis. *N Engl J Med.* 2012;367:2175-2184.

7. Hassold T, Chen N, Funkhouser J, et al. A cytogenetic study of 1000 spontaneous abortions. *Ann Hum Genet.* 1980;44:151-178.

8. Hassold T, Hall H, Hunt P. The origin of human aneuploidy: where we have been, where we are going. *Hum Mol Genet.* 2007;16(2):R203-R308.

CHAPTER

16

Molecular Diagnostic Testing

■ GENETIC MUTATIONS
■ GENETIC TESTING VERSUS GENETIC SCREENING
■ COMMONLY USED GENETIC TECHNOLOGIES
  Polymerase Chain Reaction
  Hybridization-Based Mutation Detection Techniques
  Sequencing Techniques
■ CLINICAL CONSIDERATIONS IN DIAGNOSTIC TESTING

The goal of molecular diagnostic testing is to provide definitive diagnoses for suspected or unknown genetic conditions. A precise diagnosis is important for determining what caused a particular birth defect, for making an accurate cancer diagnosis, for assessing predisposition to adult disorders, or for providing potential therapeutic targets for present and future treatments. There are dozens of molecular-genetic techniques that are currently utilized, all with the common purpose of determining pathologic variations in the primary nucleotide sequence in the affected subject. Clinical molecular testing can be divided into those tests that look at the sequence of a specific single gene, or a more shotgun approach where panels of genes or whole exomes/genomes are sequenced in order to identify the cause of the presenting condition. However, whole exome/genome sequencing provides the individual not only with a diagnosis that explains current symptoms, but also incidental medically actionable health information that may have significant implications for the patient and his/her family. Incidental actionable medical information includes detecting carrier status for a known mendelian disorder, finding susceptibility genes for various cancers, such as *BRCA1/BRCA2*, or discovering genetic changes that affect response to certain drugs.

■ GENETIC MUTATIONS

Most of the testing in molecular genetics has focused on region(s) of DNA that encode proteins (see Chapter 1, Figure 1-1).[1] These coding regions are called exons. The terms "mutation" and "variant" are used here interchangeably and may be **pathogenic**, **benign** or of **unknown** significance. We can interpret nucleotide variations easier if we find pathogenic mutations (pathogenic variants) that alter protein structure. On the other hand, many mutations can also occur outside of the coding regions of the gene, and these may involve regulatory components of the genome, such as promoters and enhancers, that regulate gene expression, or affect messenger RNA stability (mutations in the 5′ or 3′ untranslated gene regions, known as UTRs). Mutations can partially affect gene function by rendering a protein less efficient to perform its functions (androgen receptor mutations that cause incomplete androgen insensitivity syndrome), by completely abolishing the function of the protein (*CYP21A2* mutations that cause the classic form of congenital adrenal hyperplasia), by interfering with the function of the native protein (dominant negative mutations of fibrillin that cause Marfan syndrome), or by making the protein more active (fibroblast growth factor receptor 3 gene gain of function mutations that cause achondroplasia). Mutations can result from changes in a single nucleotide (point mutation) or multiple nucleotides (deletions, duplications, insertions). Point mutations within the coding region of the gene (exons) may have multiple consequences. It may cause no change in the amino acid (neutral or synonymous mutation and likely benign), may change amino acid (missense or nonsynonymous mutation which may or may not be pathogenic), or may introduce a stop codon (nonsense mutation which usually tend to be pathogenic). Point mutations outside of the exonic regions can affect splicing of exons, which leads to variant RNA transcripts that may encode proteins with no function. Insertions, deletions, and duplications involve a change in the number of nucleotide residues, and will change the amino acid composition of the protein, and therefore its function, or truncate the protein due to premature insertion of a stop codon. When reading a molecular genetic report that identifies a nucleotide variation that differs from the "reference genome" (a nonaffected control), it is important to determine whether such variation is pathogenic, or not. Many nucleotide variations cause nonsynonymous amino acid changes that are benign (not causing protein dysfunction). The population frequency of a particular variant can help distinguish benign from pathogenic nucleotide variation. A nucleotide variation that is rare, <0.5% in the population, is more likely to be pathogenic in an individual with a rare disorder, than variant that is present in more than 20% of the population. Other clues to whether a particular variant is pathogenic includes whether the changed amino acid is highly conserved among different species, whether the changed amino acid change is predicted to disrupt protein function, or whether the particular gene that harbors the variant makes physiologic sense from previous animal research showing the observed phenotype.

■ GENETIC TESTING VERSUS GENETIC SCREENING

Genetic testing can be used in different settings. It can either be applied to an individual with clear phenotype who seeks answers about the genetic etiology of their disease, or it can be used to screen populations for a highly prevalent condition. Cystic fibrosis has a relatively high carrier frequency (1 in 29) in the Caucasian population, making it appropriate for a population based screening program. Among Ashkenazi (Eastern European) Jews, the carrier frequency approaches 1 in 4 for at least one of 19 different diseases common in this ethnic group. Whole exome/genome sequencing blurs the distinction between diagnostic and screening testing, as the information obtained from such testing provides both diagnostic and screening information. For any genetic testing, pre- and posttest genetic counseling by a genetic counselor or genetic physician is of utmost importance. Genetic counseling should include information on the testing procedure, the possible results, the potential uncertainties in testing, and how the results may impact the patient and their family.

■ COMMONLY USED GENETIC TECHNOLOGIES

Polymerase Chain Reaction

Polymerase chain reaction (PCR) and PCR-based applications represent the most common methodologies used in genetic testing. This technology is based on the discovery that DNA polymerase from *Thermus aquaticus*, also known as *Taq* polymerase, resists high temperatures. The discovery of *Taq* polymerase led to the development of PCR (Figure 16-1). Each PCR cycle involves denaturing DNA double strands into single strands at high temperature (~95°C), annealing short region-specific oligonucleotides that bracket the region of interest, followed by extension synthesis of targeted regions using *Taq* DNA polymerase. The PCR

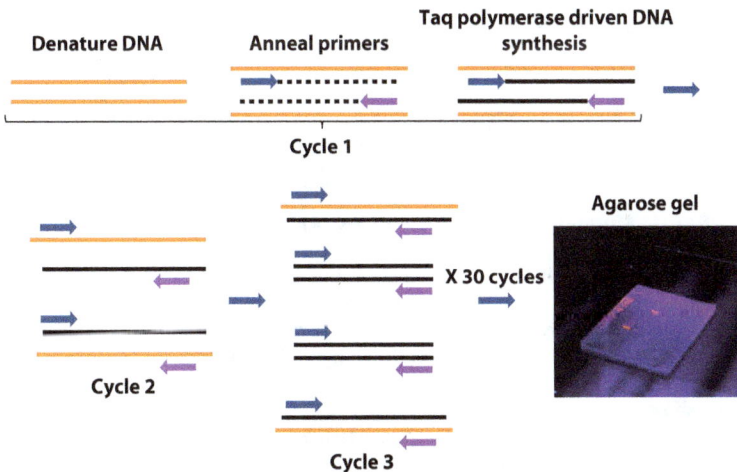

FIGURE 16-1. Polymerase chain reaction (PCR). Double-stranded DNA is initially denatured at 95°C. DNA site–specific oligonucleotides (primers) bind (anneal) to complementary single-stranded DNA derived from denatured double-stranded DNA. Taq DNA polymerase synthesizes complementary strands in the 5' to 3' direction. Each cycle consisting of DNA denaturation, annealing of primers and primer extension with Taq DNA polymerase is repeated as many times as needed to obtain the desired quantity of DNA. Agarose gel electrophoresis can be used to check on the purity of the amplified product. DNA fractionated on agarose gel and stained with ethidium bromide will fluoresce under ultraviolet light.

amplification is exponential, and creates several billion copies of uniquely targeted DNA fragments. PCR can amplify almost any genomic region with small starting amounts of DNA. It can be used to amplify all the exons within a specific gene for sequencing. Quantitative PCR is a modification of the PCR technique that quantitates the amount of DNA or RNA in the sample, and can be used to detect deletions or duplications, and determine RNA expression levels, as well as viral and bacterial loads.

Hybridization-Based Mutation Detection Techniques

The ability of complementary DNA/DNA, and DNA/RNA strands to anneal to each other is exploited by techniques based on hybridization. Hybridization to complementary DNA can be done in a variety of ways. In a dot blot, genomic DNA is not size fractionated, but bound directly to a membrane (Figure 16-2A). Short probes known as oligonucleotides (ranging from 15-21 nucleotides) are synthesized to correspond to either a wild type ("normal") allele or known pathogenic mutant allele. The probes are labeled with radioactivity and allele-specific

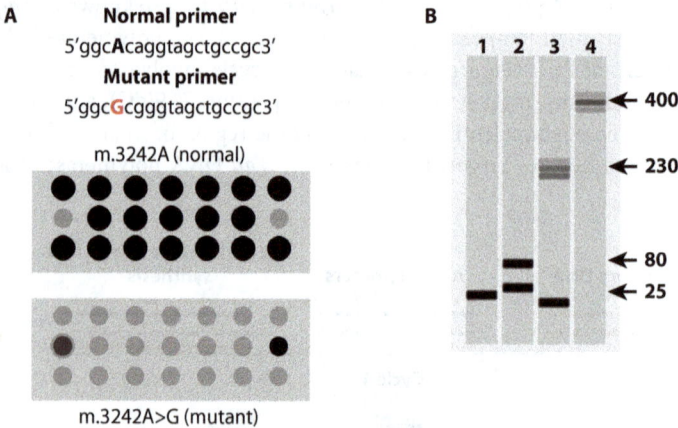

FIGURE 16-2. Mutation detection techniques. (A) Allele specific oligonucleotide based dot blot. Two sets of oligonucleotides are created, the first one detects a commonly encountered allele ("normal"), and the second one corresponds to a specific pathogenic mutant allele, known to result in pathology (change from A to G, indicated in bold and red). The top dot blot shows hybridization with a "normal" probe against 21 different clinical samples and the bottom dot blot shows hybridization of the same clinical samples with a probe that carries the mitochondrial MELAS pathogenic mutation 3243A>G. Two samples show a weak signal with the "normal" probe in the upper panel, but strong signal with a mutant probe in a lower panel, consistent with a pathogenic mutation in those two samples. **(B)** Southern blot. Lanes 1 to 4 represent four different individuals tested for fragile X CGG repeat expansion. Genomic DNA from each sample is digested with a restriction enzyme, run on agarose gel and transferred to a DNA binding membrane. The membrane is then incubated with a radioactive probe that will detect the fragile X CGG repeat containing fragment(s). Lane 1: a normal male who carries approximately 25 CGG repeats (males have a single X chromosome, hence single band), lane 2: a normal female that has normal (lower band) and expanded premutation allele (higher band, 80 CGG repeats), lane 3: an affected female has one normal and one full mutation allele (230 CGG repeats), lane 4: an affected male with one full mutation allele (400 CGG repeats).

oligonucleotide (ASO) hybridization can show a simple presence or absence of a specific pathogenic mutation in the clinical sample (Figure 16-2A).

If DNA is sorted by size using gel-electrophoresis prior to hybridization, the technique is called Southern blot hybridization (Figure 16-2B). Unlike the dot blot hybridization, the Southern blot allows determination of the size of the targeted region, and is very useful in detecting FMR1 repeats (Figure 16-2B). To detect the size of FMR1 repeats, the DNA is digested with a restriction enzyme, size fractionated by gel electrophoresis, and hybridized to a radioactive probe that is complementary to that region. Males have a single X chromosome and only one band will be visible (Lane 1, Figure 16-2B), while females carry two X chromosomes, and two bands will be visible (Lane 2, Figure 16-2B), if each allele is of a different size. FMR1 repeats in individuals with a full mutation may consist of several thousand repeats, and PCR-based techniques amplify such large repeat regions with difficulty. Therefore, Southern blot is the preferred diagnostic technique.

Other techniques that currently utilize hybridization include microarray screening for SNPs (single nucleotide polymorphisms), CGH (comparative genome hybridization) based arrays to detect genomic imbalances, and fluorescence *in situ* hybridization (see Chapter 15).

Sequencing Techniques

The gold standard in determining the primary nucleotide sequence remains Sanger sequencing. Sanger sequencing is used to sequence a single gene or individual exons. It is based on *in vitro* DNA replication in the presence of DNA polymerase and chain-terminating dideoxynucleotides with fluorochromes. A ladder of fragments differing by one nucleotide is created that can be ordered via capillary electrophoresis, and detected using laser to give the sequence of nucleotides (Figure 16-3). In reproductive genetics, Sanger sequencing is useful to identify disease causing pathogenic mutations in embryos at risk (Figure 16-4), as well as to sequence specific genes such as *BRCA1* and *BRCA2* in individuals at risk for breast and ovarian cancer syndromes. Gene panels that test multiple genes are useful in disorders such as deafness, blindness, and cardiomyopathy, as well as for ethnic disorders, such as Jewish diseases.

In many patients, the clinical presentation is compelling for a genetic disorder, but either single candidate gene testing or panel testing yields negative results. Whole exome sequencing (Figure 16-5) improves diagnostic yield in many of these undiagnosed genetic disorders by capturing and sequencing the exons of the 20,000 known protein coding human genes. A single experiment generates large amounts of data, approximately 13 billion base pairs (Gb) of sequence, and requires special programs to analyze. Each individual harbors more than a thousand unique variants, and determining whether a particular nucleotide change is pathogenic or benign can be challenging. The criteria to differentiate pathogenic from benign variants have been described earlier. In addition to those criteria, it is necessary to determine if the variant segregates with affected family members. Therefore, the larger the number of family members who participate in whole exome sequencing, the better is the success in identifying the pathogenic mutation.

A

C C A A A T T T A C A G

B

T A T G A C **A** C T C G G

G

C

C A T T C T T C A A T

C A T T C T T T C T T C A A T

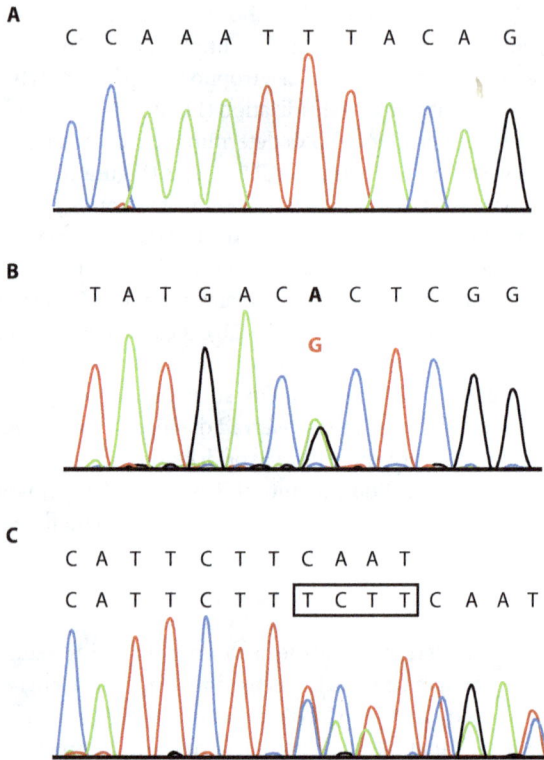

FIGURE 16-3. Sanger sequencing chromatograms. (A) Chromatogram of double stranded DNA sequence is shown. Red peaks are thymines (T), blue peaks are cytosines (C), green peaks are adenines (A), and black peaks are guanines (G). **(B)** Chromatogram of sequence with heterozygous single nucleotide polymorphism, where one allele is A and second allele is G. **(C)** Chromatogram shows a 4-bp deletion of the TCTT sequence on one allele. The deletion causes a frame shift in the sequence which can lead to a premature stop codon, or dysfunctional protein due to a change in amino acid sequence downstream from the deletion.

Sanger sequencing should be used to corroborate nucleotide variants identified by whole exome sequencing because whole exome sequencing has some limitations. Capture of some exons may fail, or coverage of some regions may not be adequate to make appropriate variant calls. Despite the potential technical limitations, whole exome sequencing allows a diagnosis to be achieved in approximately 25% of individuals that were previously undiagnosed.[2] Whole exome sequencing also may provide more personalized cancer treatments. It is possible to compare whole exome genetic variation between an individual's tumor specimen and surrounding normal tissue to identify pathogenic mutations that drive their cancer. Identification of pathogenic mutations that drive tumorigenesis may allow for more rational chemotherapy approaches and potentially better outcomes.

Whole genome sequencing refers to the sequencing of both coding (exons) and noncoding regions of the genome. Because whole exome sequencing captures only 1% of the genome, additional information obtained on whole genome

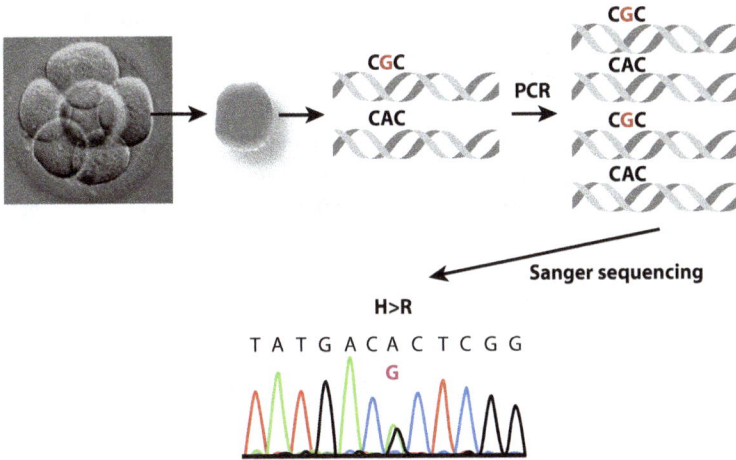

FIGURE 16-4. Preimplantation genetic diagnosis (PGD). PGD has several important steps: *in vitro* fertilization, *in vitro* culturing of early embryos, aspiration of one to two embryonic cells, DNA isolation from aspirated cells, PCR of the genomic region(s) where pathogenic mutations are to be identified and DNA sequencing. In this case, the fetus is heterozygous for a pathogenic mutation that causes adenine (A) to change to guanine (G) and changes the amino acid histidine (H) to arginine (R).

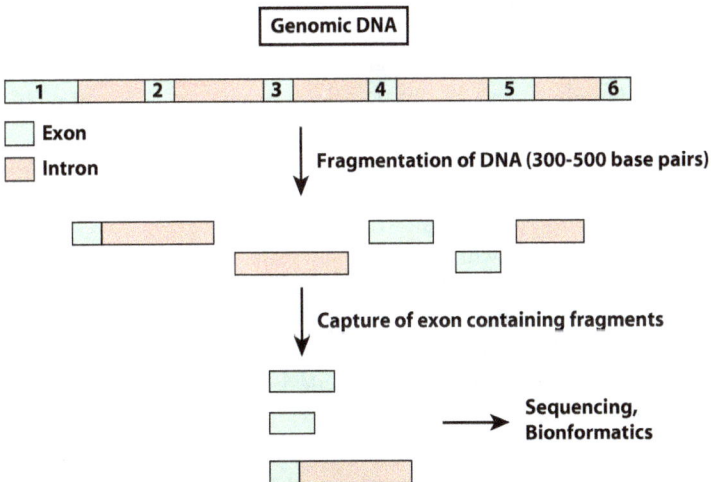

FIGURE 16-5. Whole exome sequencing. In whole exome sequencing, genomic DNA is fragmented, and specially designed baits are used to capture fragments of DNA that contain exons. Exons constitute only 1% of genomic DNA. The exon containing fragments are eluted, amplified by PCR and sequenced. Large amounts of data are generated and require specialized programs to align the sequences against the reference genome, to determine nucleotide variants that differ from the reference, and to identify pathogenic mutations.

sequencing will improve diagnostic yield. Whole genome sequencing can determine the sequence of noncoding regulatory regions that cause disease, and can determine copy number variation (not possible on whole exome sequencing due to variable capture). The disadvantages of whole genomic sequencing are the cost and difficulty in interpreting genetic variation in noncoding regions. Nonetheless, whole genome sequencing eventually will replace whole exome sequencing, and will become an essential part of the patient's medical information. These genomic approaches will allow personalized medical advice, and individualized treatment approaches.

■ CLINICAL CONSIDERATIONS IN DIAGNOSTIC TESTING

The clinical presentation should guide whether to order a specific gene test, a gene panel, or whole exome/genome sequencing. For example, an individual with a strong family history of Marfan syndrome, and clinical findings consistent with Marfan syndrome would benefit from sequencing of the fibrillin gene. For a woman whose relative has a known *BRCA1* pathogenic mutation, the genetic testing should focus on whether she inherited the particular pathogenic mutation found in the family. In individuals with multiple congenital anomalies, the first line test should be a SNP/oligonucleotide based microarray to rule out large genomic imbalances (Chapter 15). The diagnostic yield will be 25%. If the SNP/oligonucleotide microarray is normal, whole exome sequencing on the parents, and the affected individual may provide an additional 25% diagnostic yield. Including relatives in whole exome sequencing allows the exclusion of many benign rare variants that may be mistaken for pathologic variants. Many of the genetic etiologies in individuals with multiple congenital anomalies are not inherited, but *de novo*. *De novo* pathogenic mutations may be present in as many as 80% of individuals with autosomal dominant disorders, and up to 40% of individuals with X linked disorders.[2]

The question may arise as to whether to order a gene panel, or whole exome sequencing. A genetic panel for known pathogenic mutations causing cardiomyopathy is best in a woman who presents with familial cardiomyopathy. Whole exome sequencing will discover many variants of unknown significance and thus may be uninterpretable. Nonetheless, the future belongs to whole exome/genome sequencing, and a DNA profile will be an essential part of individual's medical data. It will be used by various specialists to determine disease susceptibilities, carrier status for various genetic disorders, and potential responses to therapy and medications.

REFERENCES

1. ACOG technology assessment. Genetics and molecular diagnostic testing.Number 1, July 2002. American College of Obstetrics and Gynecology. *Int J Gynaecol Obstet.* 2002;79:67-85.

2. Yang, Y., Muzny DM, Reid JG, *et al.* Clinical whole-exome sequencing for the diagnosis of mendelian disorders. *N Engl J Med.* 2013;369:1502-1511.

Index

Note: Page references followed by *f* indicate figures; those followed by *t* indicate tables.

www.ingramcontent.com/pod-product-compliance
Lightning Source LLC
Chambersburg PA
CBHW070719220326
41598CB00024BA/3231